MW01166613

POCKET REFERENCE

FOR

BLS PROVIDERS

THIRD EDITION

Bob Elling, MPA, REMT-P

PEARSON
Prentice
Hall

Upper Saddle River, New Jersey 07458

A Cataloging-in-Publication record for this book is available from the Library of Congress

Brady's *Pocket Reference for BLS Providers* was designed to provide you with a handy, pocket-size guide to which you can quickly refer.

© 2007 Pearson Education, Inc.
Upper Saddle River, New Jersey 07458

Printed in the United States of America

10 9 8 7 6 5 4 3 2 1

ISBN 0-13-173730-9

Studentaid.ed.gov, the U.S. Department of Education's website on college planning assistance, is a valuable tool for anyone intending to pursue higher education. Designed to help students at all stages of schooling, including international students, returning students, and parents, it is a guide to the financial aid process. The website presents information on applying to an attending college as well as on funding your education and paying loans. It also provides links to useful resources, such as state education agency contact information, assistance in filling out financial aid forms, and an introduction to various forms of student aid.

Dedicated to my wife Kirsten and my daughters Laura and Caitlin. May you always maintain humility as your accomplishments meet the stars.

It is the intent of the author and publisher that this reference be used as part of a formal BLS education program taught by qualified instructors and supervised by a licensed physician. The procedures described in this reference are based on consultation with EMT and medical authorities. The author and publisher have taken care to make certain that these procedures reflect currently accepted clinical practice; however, they cannot be considered absolute recommendations.

The material in this reference contains the most current information available at the time of publication. However, federal, state, and local guidelines concerning clinical practices, including, without limitation, those governing infection control and body substance isolation precautions, change rapidly. The reader should note, therefore, that the new regulations may require changes in some procedures.

It is the responsibility of the reader to familiarize himself or herself with the policies and procedures set by federal, state, and local agencies as well as the institution or agency where the reader is employed. The author and the publisher of this reference disclaim any liability, loss, or risk resulting directly or indirectly from the suggested procedures and theory, from any undetected errors, or from the reader's misunderstanding of the reference. It is the reader's responsibility to stay informed of any new changes or recommendations made by any federal, state, and local agency as well as by his or her employing institution or agency.

Contents

Contents

Assessment Skills   55

Contents

Contents

Contents

Contents

Contents

Contents

Contents

Reviewers

I would like to thank Joseph E. Byrne, Earl L. Evans, and Laura L. Walker for their review of the third edition of this pocket reference. They offered significant contributions to the improvement of this guide, and I greatly appreciate their assistance.

Joseph E. Byrne, EMT-P, IT
Director, Training and Education
Warren County Emergency Medical Services
Warren, PA

Earl L. Evans, EMT-P
EMT Instructor, Town of Colonie EMS
EMT Lab Instructor, Hudson Valley Community
    College
Paramedic, Town of Colonie EMS
EMS Director, Pepsi Arena EMS, Albany, NY
Retired Executive Director, Regional Emergency
    Medical Organization (REMO), Albany, NY

Laura L. Walker, NREMT-P, DM
Tidewater EMS Regional Council, Inc.
Norfolk, VA

Bob Elling, MPA, REMT-P, is a Professor of Management at the Andrew Jackson University, a faculty member at Hudson Valley Community College Institute of Prehospital Emergency Medicine, and a paramedic with the Town of Colonie and with the Times Union Center. Bob has served as a paramedic and Lieutenant for NYC*EMS, as Associate Director of the New York State EMS Program, as Education Coordinator for *PULSE: Emergency Medical Update,* and as BLS Guidelines 2005 editor/writer.

NORMAL RESPIRATORY RATES (BREATHS PER MINUTE, AT REST)	
Adult	12–20
Adolescent (11–14)	12–20
School age (6–10)	16–30
Preschooler (3–5)	20–30
Toddler (1–3)	20–30
Infant (6–12 months)	20–30
Infant (0–5 months)	25–40
Newborn	30–60

➤ NORMAL RESPIRATORY RHYTHM

Regular.

➤ NORMAL RESPIRATORY QUALITY

Breath sounds are present and equal.

Chest expansion is adequate and equal.

Breathing takes minimum effort.

➤ NORMAL RESPIRATORY DEPTH

Adequate.

➤ RESPIRATORY SOUNDS/POSSIBLE CAUSES

Snoring—airway partially blocked.

Wheezing—asthma, anaphylaxis.

Gurgling—fluids in the airway.

Crowing—croup.

➤ RESPIRATORY IRREGULARITIES

Breath sounds—diminished, unequal, absent.

Chest expansion—inadequate or unequal.

Effort of breathing—labored, increased respiratory effort, accessory muscle use (may be pronounced in infants/children and involve nasal flaring, seesaw breathing, grunting, and retractions between ribs and above clavicles and sternum).

NORMAL PULSE RATES (BEATS PER MINUTE, AT REST)	
Adult	60–100
Adolescent (11–14)	60–105
School age (6–10)	70–110
Preschooler (3–5)	80–120
Toddler (1–3)	80–130
Infant (6–12 months)	80–140
Infant (0–5 months)	90–140
Newborn	120–160

➤ PULSE IRREGULARITIES/POSSIBLE CAUSES

Rapid, regular, and full—exertion, fright, drugs, high blood pressure, first-stage blood loss.

Rapid, regular, and thready—shock, later stages of blood loss.

Slow—head injury, drugs, some poisons, some heart problems, hypoxia in children, well-conditioned athletes, hypothermia.

No pulse—cardiac arrest.

NORMAL BLOOD PRESSURE

	Systolic	Diastolic
Adults	90–140	60–90
Infants/children	$80 + 2 \times$ age (years)	⅔ systolic
Adolescent	88–140	(Average 59)
School age	80–122	(Average 57)
Preschooler	78–116	(Average 55)

➤ BLOOD PRESSURE IRREGULARITIES/POSSIBLE CAUSES

High blood pressure—medical condition, exertion, fright, stress, emotional distress, excitement.

Low blood pressure—athlete or other person with normally low blood pressure, blood loss, late sign of shock.

➤ SKIN COLOR

Pink—normal in light-skinned patients; normal at inner eyelids, lips, and nailbeds of dark-skinned patients.

Pale—constricted blood vessels possibly resulting from blood loss, shock, hypotension, or emotional distress.

Cyanotic—lack of oxygen resulting from inadequate breathing or heart function.

Flushed—heat exposure, high blood pressure, emotional excitement.

Jaundiced (yellow)—abnormalities of the liver.

Mottling—occasionally in patients in shock.

➤ SKIN TEMPERATURE AND CONDITION

Cool, clammy—sign of shock.

Cold, moist—body is losing heat.

Cold, dry—exposure to cold.

Hot, dry—high fever, heat exposure.

Hot, moist—high fever, heat exposure.

**"Goose pimples" with shivering, chattering teeth, blue
lips, and pale skin**—chills, exposure to cold,
communicable disease, pain, fever.

➤ PUPIL IRREGULARITIES/POSSIBLE CAUSES

Dilated—fright, blood loss, drugs (e.g., atropine),
treatment with eye drops.

Constricted—drugs (narcotics), treatment with eye
drops.

Unequal—stroke, head injury, eye injury, artificial eye.

Lack of reactivity—drugs, lack of oxygen to brain.

➤ **PUPIL GAUGE**

➤ **PAIN SCALE**

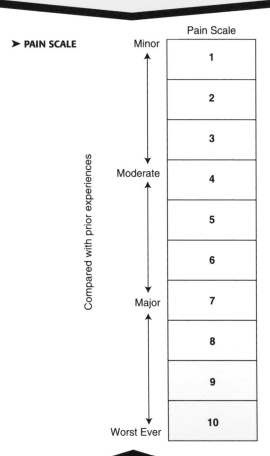

Pain Scale

	Pain Scale
Minor	1
	2
	3
Moderate	4
	5
	6
Major	7
	8
	9
Worst Ever	10

Compared with prior experiences

➤ **FLOW CHARTS**
Scene Size-up

Trauma Patient Assessment

Medical Patient Assessment

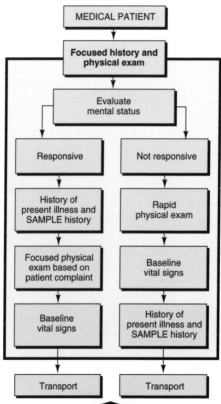

➤ SCALES, ACRONYMS, AND MNEMONICS

Mental Status: AVPU

A—Alert. Awake and oriented (person, place, day).

V—Verbal. Responds to verbal stimulus.

P—Painful. Responds to painful stimulus.

U—Unresponsive. Does not respond to any stimulus.

GLASGOW COMA SCALE		
Eye opening	Spontaneous	4
	To voice	3
	To pain	2
	None	1
Verbal responses	Oriented	5
	Inappropriate words	4
	Incomprehensible	3
	Sounds	2
	None	1
Motor response	Obeys commands	6
	Localizes pain	5
	Withdraw (pain)	4
	Flexion (pain)	3
	Extension (pain)	2
	None	1
Glasgow Coma Scale	Total	

NOTE: During the initial assessment, AVPU is used for the quick neurological exam. During the focused physical exam, the Glasgow Coma Scale (GCS) may be used for evaluating head-injured patients.

REVISED TRAUMA SCORE

Characteristic	Criterion	RTS Points	
Glasgow Coma Scale	13–15	4	
	6–12	3	
	6–8	2	
	4–5	1	
	3	0	
Systolic Blood Pressure	>89 mmHg	4	
	76–89 mmHg	3	
	50–75 mmHg	2	
	1–49 mmHg	1	
	0	0	
Respiratory Rate	10–29/min	4	
	>29/min	3	
	6–9/min	2	
	1–5/min	1	
	0	0	
Revised Trauma Score	(Total)		

Source: Champion HR, Sacco WJ, Copes WS, et. al. A Revision of the Trauma Score. J Trauma 29 (5): 623-9, 1989

OPQRRRST Questions

O—Onset. How did it start? What were you doing?

P—Provokes. Does anything make it better or worse?

Q—Quality. Can you describe it for me?

R—Radiation/Region/Referral. Where exactly is the pain? Does it seem to spread anywhere, or does it stay right there?

S—Severity. Are you uncomfortable? How bad is the pain on a scale of 1 to 10? (See Pain Scale, page 24.)

T—Time. When did the pain start? Has it changed at all since it started?

SAMPLE History

S—Signs/symptoms. Have you had any other symptoms?

A—Allergies. Are you allergic to anything?

M—Medications. What medicines do you take, and why? (OTC, prescription, herbal, recreational)

P—Pertinent past history. Do you have any other medical problems? Have you ever had this kind of problem before? Who is your doctor?

L—Last oral intake. When was the last time you ate or drank anything? What did you eat or drink?

E—Events leading to the illness. How have you felt today? Anything out of the ordinary?

DCAP-BTLS

D—Deformities.

C—Contusions.

A—Abrasions.

P—Punctures/penetrations (paradoxical motion).

B—Burns.

T—Tenderness.

L—Lacerations.

S—Swelling.

High-Priority Conditions

- Poor general impression.
- Unresponsive.
- Responsive, but not following commands.
- Difficulty breathing.
- Shock/hypoperfusion.
- Complicated childbirth.
- Chest pain with systolic blood pressure less than 100.
- Uncontrolled bleeding.
- Severe pain anywhere.

Significant Mechanisms of Injury (MOI)

- Ejection from vehicle.
- Death in same passenger compartment.
- Falls of more than 15 feet or three times the patient's height.

(continued)

- Rollover of vehicle with unrestrained occupants.
- High-speed vehicle collision.
- Vehicle–pedestrian collision.
- Motorcycle crash.
- Unresponsiveness or altered mental status.
- Penetrations of the head, chest, or abdomen.

NORMAL ADULT LAB VALUES	
Substance/Electrolyte	**Range**
Bilirubin	0.1 to 1.0 mg/dL
Calcium	8.4 to 11 mg/dL
Cholesterol	140 to 250 mg/dL
Creatinine	0.5 to 1.2 mg/dL
Sodium	135 to 147 mEq/L
Chloride	95 to 105 mEq/L
Potassium	3.5 to 5.0 mEq/L
Arterial (room air) pO_2	75 to 105 mmHg
Arterial (room air) pCO_2	33 to 44 mmHg
pH	7.35 to 7.45
Glucose (fasting)	70 to 110 mg/dL

➤ 1—HEAD TILT–CHIN LIFT MANEUVER

- Take BSI (body substance isolation) precautions.

- Once the patient is supine, place one hand on the forehead. Place the fingertips of your other hand under the bony area at the center of patient's lower jaw.

- Tilt the head by applying gentle pressure to patient's forehead.

- Use your fingertips to lift chin and to support lower jaw. Move jaw forward to a point where lower teeth are almost touching upper teeth. Do not compress soft tissues under lower jaw.

- Do not close the patient's mouth. It is best to insert an oropharyngeal airway if the patient has no gag reflex.

➤ 2—JAW-THRUST MANEUVER

- Take BSI precautions.
- Carefully keep the patient's head, neck, and spine aligned. Move the patient as a unit as you place him or her in a supine position.
- Then kneel approximately 18 inches above the head of the supine patient.
- Reach forward and gently place one hand on each side of patient's lower jaw. Run your fingers along the jaw until you just pass the angle of the jaw.
- Stabilize the patient's head with your palms and forearms.
- Using your index fingers, push the angles of the patient's lower jaw forward.
- To keep the mouth open, use an oropharyngeal airway on a patient with no gag reflex.
- Do not tilt or rotate the patient's head.

NOTE: *Remember the purpose of jaw-thrust maneuver is to open the airway without moving the head or neck from a neutral position.*

➤ 3—OROPHARYNGEAL SUCTIONING

• Take BSI precautions.

• Position yourself at patient's head, and turn patient onto his or her side, unless trauma is suspected; then leave supine.

• A rigid tip (Yankauer) is preferred. When inserting, never lose sight of the tip.

• Measure a flexible suction catheter (distance between patient's ear lobe and corner of mouth, or center of mouth to angle of jaw).

• Turn suction unit on. Attach the catheter and test for suction.

• Open and clear the patient's mouth.

• Place the rigid pharyngeal tip so that the convex (bulging-out) side is against the roof of the patient's mouth. Insert tip just to the base of the tongue. Do not push tip down into the throat or larynx.

• Apply suction only after the tip of the catheter or rigid tip is in place, suctioning on the way out, moving tip from side to side. Suction for no longer than 15 seconds. (As per U.S. DOT, suction toddlers for no longer than 10 seconds and infants for no longer than 5 seconds.)

• Ventilate the patient with 100 percent oxygen.

➤ 4—MOUTH-TO-MASK WITH OXYGEN

- Take BSI precautions.
- Connect one-way valve to mask.
- Connect oxygen to inlet on face mask. Oxygen should be run at 15 lpm.
- Kneel about 18 inches above the head of the supine patient.
- Open the airway (manually or with adjunct).
- Position mask on patient's face so that the apex is over bridge of nose and the base is between lower lip and prominence of chin.
- Use ring and middle fingers to bring patient's jaw up to mask and maintain head-tilt/chin-lift. *Tilt the head back as if you were trying to stand patient on his or her head!*
- Ventilate patient over 1 second to achieve visible chest rise.
- Remove your mouth from port to allow for passive exhalation.

NOTE: *Do not delay mouth-to-mask ventilation if oxygen is not immediately available.*

➤ 5—OROPHARYNGEAL (ORAL) AIRWAY INSERTION

- Take BSI precautions.
- Select appropriate size airway.
- Measure airway (center of mouth to angle of jaw, or corner of mouth to tip of ear lobe).
- Insert airway without pushing tongue back into throat. Insert upside down and flip 180 degrees over tongue, or insert straight in with a tongue blade holding tongue forward.
- Remove oropharyngeal airway quickly if patient gags.

➤ 6—NASOPHARYNGEAL (NASAL) AIRWAY INSERTION

- Take BSI precautions.
- Select appropriate size airway (diameter of patient's little finger). An alternative method is to measure length from patient's nostril to earlobe or to angle of jaw.
- Measure airway (nostril to ear lobe).
- Lubricate nasopharyngeal airway with water-soluble gel (e.g., KY®, Surgilube®, Lubifax®).
- Fully insert airway with bevel facing nasal septum.

➤ 7—TWO-RESCUER BAG-MASK VENTILATION

- Take BSI precautions.
- Open the medical patient's airway using head-tilt/chin-lift maneuver.
- Suction and insert an oropharyngeal airway.
- Select correct bag-mask size (adult, child, or infant). A pop-off valve is not acceptable!
- Kneel approximately 18 inches above the head of the supine patient.
- Position mask on patient's face so that the apex is over bridge of nose and the base is between the lower lip and prominence of chin.
- Position thumbs over top half of mask, index and middle fingers over bottom half.
- Use ring and middle fingers to bring patient's jaw up to mask and maintain head-tilt/chin-lift. *Tilt the head back as if you were trying to stand patient on his or her head!*
- The second rescuer should connect bag to mask, if not already done. While you maintain mask seal, second rescuer should squeeze the bag with two hands providing a ventilation over 1 second to achieve visible chest rise.
- The second rescuer should release pressure on the bag and let the patient exhale passively. While this occurs, the oxygen reservoir is refilling.

NOTE: This technique may be used for a trauma patient by combining a jaw-thrust maneuver with manual stabilization of the head and neck.

➤ 8—PREPARING OXYGEN DELIVERY SYSTEM

- Select desired cylinder. Check label and hydrostat date.
- Place cylinder in an upright position and stand to one side.
- Remove plastic wrapper or cap protecting cylinder outlet.
- Keep plastic washer (some setups).
- Crack main valve for 1 second to clean it out.
- Select correct pressure regulator and flowmeter.
- Place cylinder valve gasket on regulator oxygen port.
- Make certain that pressure regulator is closed.
- Align pins, or thread by hand.
- Tighten T-screw for pin yoke.
- Tighten with a wrench for a threaded outlet.
- Attach tubing and delivery device.

OXYGEN CYLINDER SIZES

D cylinder—contains 350 liters.
E cylinder—contains 625 liters.
M cylinder—contains 3,000 liters.
G cylinder—contains 5,300 liters.
H cylinder—contains 6,900 liters.

➤ 9—OXYGEN ADMINISTRATION VIA NONREBREATHER MASK

- Take BSI precautions.
- Assemble regulator onto tank.
- Open main valve on tank.
- Check for leaks.
- Check tank pressure.
- Attach nonrebreather mask.
- Adjust liter flow to 12 to 15 lpm.
- Pre-fill reservoir.
- Apply and adjust mask to patient's face, explaining need for oxygen.
- Secure tank during transport.

➤ 10—OXYGEN ADMINISTRATION VIA NASAL CANNULA

- Take BSI precautions.
- Assemble regulator onto tank.
- Open main valve on tank.
- Check for leaks.
- Check tank pressure.
- Attach nasal cannula to regulator.
- Place nasal prongs into the patient's nose and adjust tubing for patient comfort.
- Adjust liter flow to 1–6 lpm.
- Secure tank during transport.

➤ 11—DISCONTINUING OXYGEN ADMINISTRATION

- Remove delivery device from patient.
- Turn off the liter flow rate.
- Close the main valve.
- Remove the delivery tubing.
- Bleed the flowmeter.
- Change the tank if volume is 200 psi or less.

➤ 12—INSERTION OF ESOPHAGEAL TRACHEAL COMBITUBE® (EMT-B SKILL)

- Take BSI precautions.
- Position yourself at the patient's head.
- Assemble equipment.
- Insert the device blindly, watching for two black rings used for measuring depth of insertion. The teeth or their bony cavities, if teeth are missing, should be positioned between these rings.
- Use the large syringe to inflate the pharyngeal cuff with 100 cc of air. On inflation, the device will seat itself in the posterior pharynx behind the hard palate.
- Use the smaller syringe to fill the distal cuff with 10 cc to 15 cc of air.
- Usually (90–95 percent of the time), the tube will have been placed in the esophagus. On this assumption, ventilate through the esophageal connector (the external tube that is the longer of the two and is marked #1). You must listen for the presence of breath sounds in the lungs and the absence of sounds from the epigastrium in order to be sure that the tube is, in fact, placed in the esophagus.
- If there is an absence of lung sounds and presence of sounds in the epigastrium, the tube has been placed in the trachea. In this case, change the ventilator to the shorter tracheal connector, which is marked #2.

(continued)

- Listen again to be sure of proper placement of the tube.

➤ COMBITUBE® IN PLACE

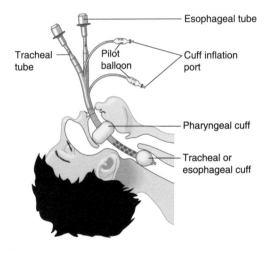

Esophageal tube

Tracheal tube

Pilot balloon

Cuff inflation port

Pharyngeal cuff

Tracheal or esophageal cuff

➤ 13—INSERTION OF THE LARYNGEAL MASK AIRWAY (LMA)® (OPTIONAL EMT-B SKILL)

- Ensure that AHA BLS (American Heart Association Basic Life Support) airway maneuvers are being attempted while preparing equipment.
- Take BSI precautions.
- Select and assemble correct equipment:
  - An LMA® properly sized for patient.
  - Bag mask with reservoir.
  - 30 cc syringe.
  - Suction unit and rigid Yankauer tip.
  - Test cuff by inflation and deflation.
  - Water-based lubricant gel for mask tip.
  - Gloves, mask, and protective eyewear.
- Have another rescuer oxygenate the patient with a bag mask.
- Place LMA®.
  - Gently introduce into oropharynx, following curvature of tube.
  - Swing mask into place in a single circular movement, ensuring pressure is maintained against palate and posterior pharynx.
  - Inflate mask without holding the tube.
  - Oxygenate the patient with the bag mask.
- Confirm LMA® placement.
  - Visually confirm chest rise.

(continued)

- - Auscultate epigastrium for absence of breath sounds.
  - Auscultate lung fields for presence of bilateral breath sounds.
  - Monitor $EtCO_2$.
- Properly secure the LMA® with tape and a bite block.
- Reassess the patient.
  - Confirm placement after LMA® is secured.
  - Reassess the ventilations for adequacy and depth.
- Document the procedure for PCR, confirming placement of the LMA® and the number of attempts.

(a) (b)

(a) Inserting the laryngeal mask airway. (b) The laryngeal mask airway in place.

➤ 14—ET INTUBATION AND MANAGEMENT (EMT-B SKILL)

- Take BSI precautions.
- Open airway manually.
- Elevate tongue and insert airway adjunct (oropharyngeal or nasopharyngeal airway).
- Ventilate patient immediately using a bag-mask device attached to high-concentration oxygen at the proper rate and volume.
- Direct assistant to oxygenate patient.
- Identify and select proper equipment for intubation.
- Check equipment (cuffs for leaks, laryngoscope batteries, and bulb for tightness).
- Position head properly (sniffing position).
- Insert laryngoscope blade with left hand while displacing tongue to the left.
- Elevate mandible with laryngoscope and visualize the vocal cords.
- Insert the ET and advance it to proper depth (until cuff is past vocal cords).
- Inflate cuff to proper pressure (5 cc to 10 cc of air) and disconnect syringe.
- Continue to hold onto the ET until it is secured in place.
- Direct ventilation of the patient.

(continued)

- Confirm proper placement by auscultation bilaterally and over epigastrium.*
- Secure the ET tube with a commercial tube restraint.

NOTE: *Most medical directors also require the use of an esophageal intubation detector device, pulse oximeter, colormetric end-tidal CO_2 device, or capnography to confirm proper tube placement.*

➤ 15—VENTILATING THE INTUBATED PATIENT

- Take BSI precautions.
- Position yourself at the patient's head.
- Look at the graduations on side of tube (e.g., adult male, 22 cm at teeth).
- Hold the tube against the patient's teeth with two fingers.
- Attach bag mask to oxygen regulator and ET tube.
- Ventilate at the proper rate (8 to 10 per minute if arrest) to achieve visible chest rise.
- Pay close attention to what ventilations feel like. Report any change in resistance.
- With each defibrillation attempt, carefully remove the bag from the tube.
- Watch for any change in the patient's mental status. A patient who becomes more alert may need to be physically or chemically restrained (by the paramedics) to prevent him or her from pulling out the tube.

NOTE: *Be especially careful not to disturb the ET tube. If it is pushed in, it will most likely enter the right mainstem bronchus, preventing oxygen from entering the patient's left lung. If it is pulled out, it can easily slip into the esophagus and send all ventilations directly to the stomach, denying the patient oxygen. This is a fatal complication if it goes unnoticed. The tube placement should be monitored using capnography.*

➤ 16—OROTRACHEAL SUCTIONING (EMT-B SKILL)

- Take BSI precautions (including sterile gloves).
- Position yourself at the patient's head.
- Hyperoxygenate the patient.
- Carefully check equipment.
- Grasp catheter with sterile gloved hand and connect it to the suction device.
- Stop ventilations, occlude suction, and insert catheter into ET tube.
- Catheter may be advanced as far as carina.
- Advance catheter to desired level, apply suction, and withdraw catheter with twisting motion, no more than 15 seconds for adults.
- Start ventilations, and rinse catheter in sterile solution.
- Suction again as needed.

NOTE: This is a sterile procedure throughout.

➤ 17—INSERTION OF NASOGASTRIC TUBE (EMT-B SKILL)

- Take BSI precautions.
- Prepare and assemble the equipment.
- Oxygenate the patient.

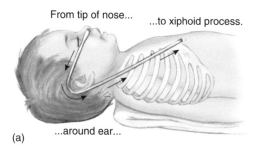

From tip of nose... ...to xiphoid process.

...around ear...

(a)

Epiglottis

Trachea

(b)

(*continued*)

- Measure tube from tip of nose, over ear, to below xiphoid process.
- Lubricate end of tube, and pass tube gently downward along nasal floor to stomach.
- To confirm correct placement, auscultate over epigastrium. Listen for bubbling while injecting 10 to 20 cc air into tube.
- Use suction to aspirate stomach contents.
- Secure tube in place.

➤ 18—USING THE PULSE OXIMETER

- Review the instruction manual for the specific unit you are using.

- Properly assemble finger-clip sensor and extension to pulse oximeter.

- Properly affix finger-clip sensor to index finger. (It may be necessary to quickly remove patient's fingernail polish.)

- Turn on pulse oximeter, and record heart and oxygen readings. Spot-check mode and extended mode (30 minutes).

- When done using oximeter, turn off the unit. After each use, disassemble and store wiring and accessories in pouch provided.

- Review operation of all display indicators, pulse amplitude, low battery, pulse search, oxygen saturation, and pulse rate.

- Review all controls (i.e., measure button, battery check button, printer on/off, printer paper advance).

- Change battery and paper printout if needed.

➤ 19—BLOOD PRESSURE BY AUSCULTATION

- Place stethoscope around your neck.
- Patient should be seated or lying down.
- If patient has not been injured, support his or her arm at heart level.
- Place cuff snugly around upper arm so that bottom of cuff is about 1 inch above crease of elbow.
- With your fingertips, palpate brachial artery at crease of elbow.
- Place the tips of stethoscope in your ears.
- Position the diaphragm of the stethoscope directly over the brachial pulse or over medial anterior elbow if no brachial pulse can be felt.
- Inflate cuff with bulb valve closed.
- Once you no longer hear brachial pulse, continue to inflate cuff until gauge reads 30 mmHg higher than the point where pulse sound disappeared.
- Slowly release air from cuff by opening bulb valve, allowing pressure to fall smoothly at rate of approximately 10 mm per second.
- When you hear the first clicking or tapping sounds, note the reading on the gauge. This is the systolic pressure.
- Continue to deflate cuff and listen for point at which these distinctive sounds fade. When sounds turn to dull, muffled thuds, the reading on gauge is the diastolic pressure.
- After obtaining diastolic pressure, let cuff deflate rapidly.

➤ 20—BLOOD PRESSURE BY PALPATION

- Find radial pulse on the arm to which blood pressure cuff is applied.

- With bulb valve closed, inflate cuff to a point where you can no longer feel the radial pulse.

- Note this point on gauge, and continue to inflate cuff until gauge reads 30 mmHg higher than point where pulse disappeared.

- Slowly deflate cuff, noting the reading at which the radial pulse returns. This reading is the systolic pressure.

- After obtaining systolic reading, let cuff deflate.

NOTE: *You cannot determine diastolic reading by palpation.*

➤ 21—INITIAL ASSESSMENT

- Take BSI precautions.
- Form a general impression based on assessment of environment and patient's chief complaint and appearance.
- Assess mental status. Determine level of responsiveness using AVPU (alert, verbal, painful, unresponsive).
- Assess airway and breathing (assess, initiate appropriate oxygen therapy, assure adequate ventilation).
- Assess circulation (assess for and control major bleeding; assess pulse; assess skin color, temperature, and condition).
- Determine patient's treatment priority (high/low, red/green) and make transport decision (unstable/stable).

NOTE: *Apply manual stabilization on first contact with any patient who you suspect may have an injury to the spine.*

➤ 22—FOCUSED HISTORY AND PHYSICAL EXAM—RESPONSIVE MEDICAL PATIENT

- Take BSI precautions.
- Gather history of current illness from patient by asking OPQRST questions.
- Gather a SAMPLE history from patient.
- Conduct a focused physical exam (focusing on the area patient complains of).
- Obtain baseline vital signs.
- Perform interventions and contact on-line medical direction as needed.
- Transport (re-evaluate transport decision).

➤ 23—FOCUSED HISTORY AND PHYSICAL EXAM—UNRESPONSIVE MEDICAL PATIENT

• Take BSI precautions.
• Conduct a rapid physical exam, by assessing:
  • Head.
  • Neck.
  • Chest.
  • Abdomen.
  • Pelvis.
  • Extremities.
  • Posterior.
• Obtain baseline vital signs.
• Gather history of the current illness from bystanders or family by asking OPQRST questions.
• Gather a SAMPLE history from bystanders or family.
• Perform interventions (obtain medical direction as required locally). Reassess vital signs.
• Transport (re-evaluate transport decision).

➤ 24—FOCUSED HISTORY AND PHYSICAL EXAM—TRAUMA PATIENT, NO SIGNIFICANT MOI

- Take BSI precautions.
- Reconsider MOI.
- Determine patient's chief complaint.
- Conduct a focused physical exam (focusing on the area patient complains of plus areas of potential injury suggested by the MOI).
- Obtain baseline vital signs.
- Take a SAMPLE history.
- Perform interventions as needed.
- Transport.

➤ 25—FOCUSED HISTORY AND PHYSICAL EXAM—TRAUMA PATIENT, SIGNIFICANT MOI

- Take BSI precautions.
- Reconsider MOI.
- Continue manual stabilization of head and neck.
- Consider requesting ALS (Advanced Life Support) personnel.
- Reconsider your transport decision.
- Reassess mental status.
- Perform a rapid trauma assessment. After assessing head and neck, apply a cervical collar and continue to maintain manual stabilization.
- Obtain baseline vital signs.
- Take a SAMPLE history.
- Perform a detailed physical exam (DCAP-BTLS) either on scene, if there is time, or en route to the hospital.
- Perform ongoing assessment, including serial vital signs.
- Transport.

➤ 26—RAPID TRAUMA ASSESSMENT

- Take BSI precautions.
- Assess head: DCAP-BTLS + crepitation.
- Assess neck: DCAP-BTLS + jugular vein distention (JVD) and crepitation.
- Assess chest: DCAP-BTLS + paradoxical motion, crepitation, breath sounds.
- Assess abdomen: DCAP-BTLS + firmness, softness, distention.
- Assess pelvis: DCAP-BTLS + pain, tenderness, motion.
- Assess extremities: DCAP-BTLS + distal pulse, motor function, and sensation.
- Assess posterior: DCAP-BTLS.

➤ 27—DETAILED PHYSICAL EXAM

- Take BSI precautions.
- Examine head: DCAP-BTLS + crepitation.
- Examine scalp and cranium: DCAP-BTLS + crepitation.
- Examine face: DCAP-BTLS.
- Examine ears: DCAP-BTLS + drainage.
- Examine eyes: DCAP-BTLS + discoloration, unequal pupils, foreign bodies, blood in anterior chamber.
- Examine nose: DCAP-BTLS + drainage, bleeding.
- Examine mouth: DCAP-BTLS + loose or broken teeth, objects that could cause obstruction, swelling or laceration of tongue, unusual breath odors, discoloration.
- Examine neck: DCAP-BTLS + jugular vein distention (JVD), crepitation.
- Examine chest: DCAP-BTLS + paradoxical motion, crepitation, breath sounds.
- Examine abdomen: DCAP-BTLS + firmness, softness, distention.
- Examine pelvis: DCAP-BTLS + pain, tenderness, motion.
- Examine extremities: DCAP-BTLS + distal pulse, motor function, sensation.
- Examine posterior: DCAP-BTLS.
- Reassess serial vital signs.

➤ 28—ONGOING ASSESSMENT

- Take BSI precautions.
- Repeat initial assessment for life threats:
  - Reassess mental status.
  - Maintain open airway.
  - Monitor breathing rate and quality.
  - Reassess pulse rate and quality.
  - Monitor skin color, temperature, and condition.
  - Re-establish patient treatment priorities.
- Reassess and record serial vital signs.
- Repeat focused assessment related to chief complaint or injuries.
- Check interventions.
  - Assure adequacy of oxygen delivery and ventilation support.
  - Assure management of bleeding.
  - Assure adequacy of interventions.

NOTE: *Repeat the ongoing assessment every 15 minutes for a stable patient; every 5 minutes for an unstable patient.*

➤ 29–CINCINNATI PREHOSPITAL STROKE SCALE

This is a very useful tool for the assessment of a patient with a suspected stroke. The AHA Guidelines 2005 recommend that all prehospital personnel be trained in its routine use. Because the care of a suspected stroke patient is "time dependent" (time is brain tissue), it is also important for the BLS Provider to be familiar with their local transport protocols and the designation of "STROKE CENTERS" as well as establishing the last time the patient was seen acting normal to start the stroke treatment clock.

EVALUATE THE FOLLOWING THREE AREAS: FACIAL DROOP, ARM DRIFT (PRONATOR DRIFT), AND SPEECH

Parameter	Normal Finding	Abnormal Finding
Facial droop	Both sides of the face move equally.	One side of the face does not move at all.
Arm (pronator) drift	Both arms move equally or not at all.	One arm drifts when compared with the other.
Speech—have them state a simple sentence	Patient uses correct words without slurring.	Slurred or inappropriate words or mute.

➤ 30—APPLYING STANDARD THREE/FOUR-LEAD ECG ELECTRODES

- Take BSI precautions.
- Turn on the ECG monitor.
- Plug in monitoring cables or leads.
- Attach monitoring cables to electrodes.
- Apply electrodes to patient's body. The most common initial configuration is lead II, which involves placing the negative lead on the right shoulder area of the chest, the ground lead on the left shoulder of the chest, and the positive lead on the left lower chest.

NOTE: In very hairy patients, it may be necessary to shave electrode attachment points on chest.

Electrode placement–frontal plane.

The standard limb leads.

➤ 31—APPLYING TWELVE-LEAD ECG ELECTRODES

- Take BSI precautions.
- Turn on the ECG monitor.
- Plug in monitoring cables or leads.
- Attach monitoring cables to electrodes. Apply electrodes to patient's body, using the following locations for each electrode.
  - *V1*—Fourth intercostal space at the right border of the sternum.

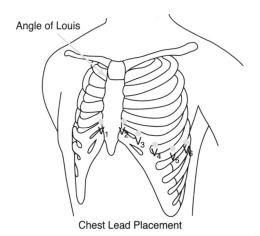

Chest Lead Placement

(*continued*)

- *V2*—Fourth intercostal space at the left border of the sternum.
- *V3*—Midway between locations V2 and V4.
- *V4*—At the mid-clavicular line in the fifth intercostal space.
- *V5*—At the anterior axillary line on the same horizontal as V4.
- *V6*—At the mid-axillary line on the same horizontal level as V4 and V5.
- *RA*—Anywhere on the right arm.
- *LA*—Anywhere on the left arm.
- *RL*—Anywhere on the right leg.
- *LL*—Anywhere on the left leg.

➤ 32—SETTING UP AND RUNNING AN IV LINE

- Take BSI precautions.
- Inspect fluid bag for clarity, expiration date, and leaks. Remove outer wrapper and gently squeeze bag.
- Verify type of solution with ALS provider.
- Select proper administration set, uncoil tubing, and keep ends sterile.
- Connect an extension set, if using a mini-drip.
- Make sure flow regulator is closed by rolling stopcock away from direction of fluid bag.
- Remove protective coverings from port of fluid bag and spiked end of tubing. Insert spiked end of tubing into fluid bag with a quick twist.
- Hold fluid bag higher than drip chamber. Squeeze drip chamber one or two times to start flow. Fill chamber marker line (one-third full).
- Open flow regulator and allow fluid to flush all air from tubing. You may need to loosen cap at lower end to get fluid flowing. *Be very careful to maintain sterility and to replace cap.*

➤ 33—USING A BLOOD GLUCOSE METER (EMT-B SKILL WITH MEDICAL DIRECTOR AUTHORIZATION)

- Take BSI precautions.

- Prepare the blood glucose meter and supplies (i.e., lancet, test strip, Band-Aid, sharps container, alcohol prep).

- Cleanse the skin with an alcohol prep. Allow the alcohol to dry before performing the finger stick.

- Use the lancet to perform a finger stick. Wipe away the first drop of blood that appears. Squeeze the finger to get a second drop of blood.

- Apply the blood to the test strip. This may be done by holding strip to the finger to draw the blood into the strip.

- Dispose of the lancet in a sharps container.

- Read the blood glucose level displayed on the glucose meter. It may take from 15 to 60 seconds for the device to provide a reading.

- Assess the puncture site and apply direct pressure or a Band-Aid to control the bleeding.

The reading is in mg/dL (milligrams of glucose per deciliter of blood). Normal "fasting" blood sugar values are 70–110 mg/dL. If the patient has a value less than 60–80 mg/dL and is symptomatic, treatment should be provided after local medical control.

➤ 34—REPOSITIONING ADULT PATIENT FOR BLS

- Take BSI precautions.
- Straighten patient's legs and position arm closest to you above his or her head.
- Cradle patient's head and neck. Grasp under the distant armpit.
- Move patient as a unit onto his or her side.
- Move patient onto back and reposition the extended arm.

NOTE: This maneuver is used to initiate airway evaluation, artificial ventilation, or CPR when rescuer must act alone. When trauma is suspected and there is ADEQUATE help, a four-rescuer log roll is the preferred technique.

➤ 35—ONE-RESCUER CPR—ADULT/CHILD PATIENT

- Check response: tap and speak loudly, "Are you all right?"
- Tell someone to call 911 and get an AED (Automated External Defibrillator).
- Open airway using the head-tilt/chin-lift.
- Check breathing (5 to 10 seconds).
- Give 2 breaths (1 second each noting visible chest rise).
- Check carotid pulse (5 to 10 seconds).
- Locate CPR hand position (center of chest between nipples).
- Deliver 30 compressions (press hard, fast [rate of 100/min] and allow full chest recoil).
- Give 2 breaths (1 second each noting visible chest rise).
- Continue cycles of 30:2 for 2 minutes (approximately 5 cycles) then reassess patient.

NOTES:
A) Depth of compression is $1\frac{1}{2}$ to 2 inches in adult and $\frac{1}{3}$ to $\frac{1}{2}$ depth of the chest in a child. A child is from 1 year to puberty.
B) Interruptions in chest compressions should be kept to a minimum and no longer than 10 seconds.
C) Once the AED arrives at the patient's side, after the first 5 cycles or 2 minutes of CPR, the following steps should be accomplished:

(continued)

- *Turn on the AED.*
- *Select pads and place pads properly.*
- *Clear patient to analyze.*
- *Clear patient to shock, press the shock button.*
- *Immediately begin CPR with compressions. If patient is going to awaken, this may take a little time to occur.*

➤ 36—TWO-RESCUER CPR—ADULT PATIENT

- Check for response.
- If no response, send someone to activate the emergency response system and get the AED.
- Open the airway using the head-tilt/chin-lift.
- Check for breathing (5 to 10 seconds).
- If no breathing, give 2 breaths (1 second each to achieve visible chest rise).
- Check carotid pulse (5 to 10 seconds).
- If no pulse, start cycles of 30 compressions to 2 breaths. Push hard and fast (100 per minute) and allow full chest recoil.
- After 5 cycles (approximately 2 minutes), if the AED has arrived apply and administer a single shock if a shockable rhythm.
- Continue CPR immediately, unless the patient wakes up.

NOTES:

A) If there are additional rescuers trained in CPR, use two rescuers to do compressions. Both should kneel on opposite sides of the patient. One does compressions for approximately 2 minutes while the other is in the ready position. Then the other rescuer should do compressions while the first rescuer takes a 2-minute break. By staying in the ready position, the switch will not take any time to interrupt compressions, and rescuer fatigue will be minimized.

B) *Minimize interruptions in compressions to less than 10 seconds.*

C) *If the patient receives an advanced airway device by an appropriately trained EMS provider, once the airway is placed the compressions will be 100 per minute and the ventilations will be 8 to 10 per minute and need not be synchronous.*

➤ 37—CHECKING THE AED

Check the AED for the following:

- Unit, cables, connectors for cleanliness.
- Supplies carried with AED.
- Power supply and its operation.
- Indicators on ECG display.
- ECG recorder operation.
- Charge display cycle with a simulator.
- Pacemaker feature, if applicable.
- File a written report on status of AED.

NOTE: This list is derived from FDA Automated Defibrillator: Operator's Shift Checklist.

➤ 38—USING THE AUTO-PULSE®

- Take BSI precautions.

- Assure CPR is in progress and effective.

- Align the patient on the Auto-Pulse® platform.

- Close the Lifeband chest band over the patient's chest.

- Press the start (Auto-Pulse® is designed to do the compressions automatically).

- Provide the bag-mask ventilation at a rate of 2 ventilations for every 30 compressions. Each ventilation should be given over 1 second to provide visible chest rise.

- If an advanced airway is in place (ETT, LMA, or Combitube), there are no longer cycles of compressions to ventilations. The compression rate is continuous 100/min and ventilation rate is 8–10/min.

- After 2 minutes of CPR, reassess for pulse and/or shockable rhythm.*

NOTE: *Always limit interruptions in chest compressions to 10 seconds or less.*

➤ 39—USING THE THUMPER®

- Take BSI precautions.
- Assure CPR is in progress and effective.
- Attach Thumper® base plate to long backboard.
- Stop CPR to slide long backboard under patient.
- Restart CPR and attach shoulder straps to patient.
- Slide Thumper® piston plate into position on base plate (away from chest).
- Stop CPR and quickly pivot piston arm into place, measuring anterior/posterior and middle sternum placement.
- Slowly adjust depth of compression to appropriate diagram.
- Adjust ventilations.
- Turn off compressions temporarily for pulse checks and defibrillation.*
- Upon termination of arrest or return of spontaneous circulation, power down unit.**

---

*NOTE: *Always limit interruptions in chest compressions to 10 seconds or less.*
*NOTE: **Always store with compression depth turned down to minimum setting.*

➤ 40—FBAO–INFANT–CONSCIOUS PATIENT

- If severe obstruction—open the airway and determine if the infant can make any sounds or breathe.
- If you are not EMS—send someone to activate the emergency response system.
- Place infant in your lap or on your knee and bare his chest.
- Holding infant prone with your forearm, deliver 5 back slaps forcefully between the infant's shoulder blades.
- Carefully turn the infant as a unit so he is resting on your forearm in a supine position.
- Provide 5 chest thrusts (CPR chest compressions) one finger's width below the nipple line.
- Repeat the series of 5 back slaps and 5 chest thrusts until object is dislodged or infant goes unconscious.

NOTES:
A) Current terminology is "mild vs. severe" airway obstruction. The BLS provider should act if signs of severe airway obstruction are observed (i.e., poor air exchange, increased breathing difficulty, a silent cough, cyanosis, or inability to speak or breathe).
B) If infant has a mild obstruction with good air exchange, forceful cough or wheeze, monitor the situation.
C) An infant is up to 1 year old, and the depth of compression is ⅓ to ½ depth of the chest.
D) When holding the infant, prone or supine, carefully tilt him slightly so fluid can drain from the mouth.

➤ 41—FBAO—INFANT—PATIENT BECOMES UNCONSCIOUS

- Kneel or sit with infant in your lap or on your knee.
- Bare the infant's chest.
- Carefully hold the infant in a prone position resting on your forearm and on your knee or lap.
- Deliver up to 5 back slaps.
- Carefully turn the infant to a supine position resting on your forearm and on your knee or lap.
- Deliver up to 5 CPR chest compressions (center of chest one finger below nipple line).
- Continue the cycles of 5 back slaps and 5 chest compressions until infant responds or becomes unconscious.
- If unconscious, place the infant on a firm flat surface.
- Open the airway and look in the mouth for an object. Do not perform a blind finger sweep. If an object is seen, remove it.
- Begin CPR with the extra step of looking in the mouth each time you open the airway, looking for the obstruction in the back of the throat. If you see it, remove it.
- After 5 cycles (approximately 2 minutes) of CPR, activate the emergency response system if you are not EMS.

(*continued*)

NOTES:
A) When reassessing the patient, look in the mouth/airway for an object that can easily be removed but do not do a blind finger sweep.
B) Depth of compression is $\frac{1}{3}$ to $\frac{1}{2}$ depth of the chest in an infant.

➤ 42—FBAO–INFANT–UNCONSCIOUS PATIENT

- If unconscious, place the infant on a firm flat surface.
- Open the airway and look in the mouth for an object. Do not perform a blind finger sweep. If an object is seen, remove it.
- Begin CPR with the extra step of looking in the mouth each time you open the airway, looking for the obstruction in the back of the throat. If you see it, remove it.
- After 5 cycles (approximately 2 minutes) of CPR, activate the emergency response system if you are not EMS.

NOTES:
A) When reassessing the patient, look in the mouth/airway for an object that can easily be removed but do not do a blind finger sweep.
B) Depth of compression is $\frac{1}{3}$ to $\frac{1}{2}$ depth of the chest in an infant.

➤ 43—FBAO–ADULT/CHILD–CONSCIOUS

- If severe obstruction—ask the patient, "Are you choking?"
- If you are not EMS—send someone to activate the emergency response system.
- Stand or kneel behind the patient and wrap your arms around them.
- Make a fist and place the thumb side of your fist against the abdomen midline slightly above the navel but below the xiphoid process.
- Grasp your fist with the other hand and thrust inward and upward.
- Repeat the abdominal thrusts until the object is expelled or the patient becomes unresponsive.

NOTES:
A) Current terminology is "mild vs. severe" airway obstruction. The BLS provider should act if signs of severe airway obstruction are observed (i.e., poor air exchange, increased breathing difficulty, a silent cough, cyanosis, or inability to speak or breathe).
B) If adult or child has a mild obstruction with good air exchange, forceful cough or wheeze, monitor the situation.
C) A child is from 1 year to puberty.
D) The depth of compression for an adult is $1\frac{1}{2}$ to 2 inches and a child is $\frac{1}{3}$ to $\frac{1}{2}$ depth of the chest.
E) For pregnant or obese patients, the chest thrust (CPR compression) should be substituted for abdominal thrusts.

Adult/Child Foreign-Body Airway
Obstruction (FBAO)

➤ 44—FBAO–ADULT/CHILD–BECOMES UNCONSCIOUS

- Carefully assist the patient to the ground/floor.
- Activate the emergency response number.
- Open the airway (head-tilt/chin-lift) and check breathing (5 to 10 seconds). If you see something in the airway, remove it. Otherwise, finger sweeps are not recommended.
- Give 2 breaths (1 second each noting visible chest rise*).
- Check carotid pulse (5 to 10 seconds).
- Locate CPR hand position (center of chest between nipples).
- Deliver 30 compressions (press hard, fast [rate of 100/min] and allow full chest recoil).
- Give 2 breaths (1 second each noting visible chest rise).
- Continue cycles of 30:2 for 2 minutes (approximately 5 cycles) then reassess patient.**
- If the obstruction clears and you can ventilate, proceed with assessment and steps of CPR. If the obstruction does not clear, continue cycles of compressions and attempts at ventilation.

NOTES:
A) * If no visible chest rise after second breath, proceed immediately to chest compressions.

(continued)

B) ** When reassessing the patient, look in the mouth/airway for an object that can easily be removed but do not do a blind finger sweep.

C) Depth of compression is 1½ to 2 inches in adult and ⅓ to ½ depth of the chest in a child. A child is from 1 year to puberty.

➤ 45—FBAO—ADULT/CHILD—UNCONSCIOUS

- Activate the emergency response number.
- Open the airway using the head-tilt/chin-lift.
- Check breathing (5 to 10 seconds).
- Gives 2 breaths (1 second each noting visible chest rise*).
- Checks carotid pulse (5 to 10 seconds).
- Locate CPR hand position (center of chest between nipples).
- Deliver 30 compressions (press hard, fast [rate of 100/min] and allow full chest recoil).
- Give 2 breaths (1 second each noting visible chest rise).
- Continue cycles of 30:2 for 2 minutes (approximately 5 cycles) then reassess patient.**

NOTES:
A) This is suspected because you may not know the patient is completely obstructed until you attempt ventilation.
B) * If no visible chest rise after second breath, proceed to chest compressions.
C) ** When reassessing the patient, look in the mouth/airway for an object that can easily be removed but do not do a blind finger sweep.

➤ 46—BLEEDING CONTROL/SHOCK MANAGEMENT

- Take BSI precautions.
- Apply direct pressure to wound.
- Elevate the extremity.
- Apply a dressing to wound.
- If wound continues to bleed, apply an additional dressing to wound. Do not remove initial layer(s).
- If wound continues to bleed, locate and apply pressure to appropriate arterial pressure point.
- For extremity profuse arterial bleeding uncontrolled by pressure point, apply an arterial tourniquet.
- Apply high-concentration oxygen.
- Properly position patient.
- Initiate steps to prevent heat loss from patient.
- Indicate need for immediate transport.

➤ 47—APPLICATION OF PASG

- Take BSI precautions.
- Assure patient meets local protocol for PASG (Pneumatic Anti-Shock Garment).
- Check for contraindications (e.g., pulmonary edema or penetrating chest injury).
- Remove clothing and check for sharp objects.
- Quickly assess areas that will be under PASG.
- Position PASG with top of abdominal section at or below last set of ribs.
- Secure PASG around patient.
- Attach hoses. Open stopcock valves.
- Check patient's blood pressure.
- Begin inflation sequence.
- Stop inflation sequence at 106 mmHg or pop-off valves release. Close stopcock valves.
- Operate PASG to maintain air pressure in device.
- Reassess patient's vital signs.

WARNING: Do not actually inflate a PASG on a mock victim in class.

NOTE: MAST (military anti-shock trousers) is another name for the PASG and is used primarily for pelvic fractures.

➤ 48—IMMOBILIZATION: LONG BONE

- Take BSI precautions.
- Direct application of manual stabilization.
- Assess distal pulses, motor ability, and sensory response (PMS).
- Measure splint.
- Apply splint.
- Immobilize injury site and joints above and below injury.
- Secure entire injured extremity from distal to proximal direction.
- Immobilize hand/foot in functional position.
- Reassess distal PMS.

➤ 49—REALIGNING AN EXTREMITY

• Take BSI precautions.

• Assess distal pulses, motor ability, and sensory response (PMS).

• Rescuer A grasps distal extremity, while Rescuer B places one hand above and below injury site.

• Rescuer B supports injury site, while Rescuer A pulls gentle manual traction in direction of long axis of body. If resistance is felt or if it appears that bone ends will come through skin, stop realignment and splint extremity in position found.

• If no resistance is felt, maintain gentle traction until extremity is properly splinted.

• Reassess distal PMS.

➤ 50—IMMOBILIZATION: JOINT INJURY

- Take BSI precautions.
- Direct application of manual stabilization of injury.
- Assess distal pulses, motor ability, and sensory response (PMS).
- Select proper splinting device.
- Immobilize the site of injury and the bones above and below.
- Reassess distal PMS.

➤ 51—IMMOBILIZATION: TRACTION SPLINT

- Take BSI precautions.
- Direct manual stabilization of injured leg.
- Assess distal pulses, motor ability, and sensory response (PMS).
- Direct application of manual traction.
- Adjust and position splint at the injured leg.
- Apply proximal securing device (e.g., ischial strap).
- Apply distal securing device (e.g., ankle hitch).
- Apply mechanical traction.
- Position and secure support straps.
- Reassess distal PMS.
- Secure patient's torso and traction splint to long backboard for transport.

➤ 52—SPINAL IMMOBILIZATION: SUPINE PATIENT

- Take BSI precautions.
- Direct assistant to place head in neutral, in-line position and to maintain manual stabilization until the patient is completely immobilized.
- Assess distal pulses, motor ability, and sensory response (PMS).
- Apply a properly sized rigid extrication collar.
- Position immobilization device appropriately.
- Move patient onto device without compromising integrity of spine. Apply padding to voids between torso and board as needed.
- Immobilize patient's torso to device.
- Evaluate and pad behind patient's head as necessary.
- Pad and immobilize patient's head.
- Secure patient's arms and legs to board.
- Reassess distal PMS.

➤ 53—SPINAL IMMOBILIZATION: SEATED PATIENT

- Take BSI precautions.
- Direct assistant to manually stabilize head in neutral, in-line position.
- Assess distal pulses, motor ability, and sensory response (PMS).
- Apply a properly sized rigid extrication collar.
- Position immobilization device behind the patient.
- Secure device to the patient's torso.
- Evaluate and pad behind head as needed.
- Secure patient's head to device.
- Evaluate and adjust straps.
- Secure wrists and legs.
- Reassess distal PMS.
- Transfer patient to long backboard.

➤ 54—RAPID EXTRICATION

Step 1: Perform an initial assessment

- **Rescuer A:** Maintain manual stabilization of patient's head and neck.
- **Rescuer B:** Conduct initial assessment of patient and determine need for rapid extrication based on patient status. Assess pulses, motor ability, and sensory response (PMS) in four extremities.

Step 2: Apply a cervical collar

- **Rescuer B:** Apply a properly sized cervical collar.
- **Rescuer A:** Continue to maintain manual stabilization before, during, and after application of collar.

Step 3: Lift patient and position the long backboard

- **Rescuer B:** Hold patient's armpit, and join hands with Rescuer C under patient's thighs.
- **Rescuer A:** Call for a lift while maintaining manual stabilization.
- **Rescuer B:** Lift patient approximately 2 inches off seat with Rescuer C.
- **Bystander (or fourth rescuer):** Insert long backboard under patient on seat.

Step 4: Begin to position patient for extrication

- **Rescuer B:** Reach across patient's chest and support by both armpits.
- **Rescuer A:** While maintaining manual stabilization, call for one-fourth turn, so patient is moved perpendicular to steering wheel, ready to exit car head first. *(continued)*

- *Rescuer C:* Free patient's lower legs from any obstructions.
- *Rescuer B:* Begin to turn patient's back toward door until Rescuer A says "stop turn."
- *Rescuer A:* Turn patient. Call for "stop turn" just before being unable to hold patient's head anymore.
- *Rescuer C:* Begin to turn patient's back toward door, freeing legs, then sliding up to thighs until Rescuer A says "stop."

Step 5: Complete another one-fourth turn

- *Rescuer B:* Stop move and wait for Rescuer C. Then take over manual stabilization of head and neck from Rescuer A.
- *Rescuer A:* Maintain head/neck stabilization until Rescuer B takes over, allowing him or her to either exit car and work from outside or reach over seat from inside if there is room or if roof has been removed.
- *Rescuer C:* Move hands from thighs to patient's armpits. Then replace Rescuer B.
- *Rescuers A, B, and C:* Complete another one-fourth turn.

Step 6: Lower patient onto the long backboard

- *Rescuer B:* Lower patient onto long backboard.
- *Rescuer A:* Call for move to lower patient's torso into a supine position on the long backboard.
- *Rescuer C:* Lower patient onto long backboard.
- *Bystander (or fourth rescuer):* Stabilize the board.

(continued)

Step 7: Position patient on the backboard

- *Rescuer B:* Slide patient as a unit.
- *Rescuer A:* Call for move to slide patient toward head end of backboard. Once in position, tell partners to "stop." Slide chest as a unit.
- *Rescuer C:* Slide pelvis as a unit until Rescuer A says "stop."
- *Bystander (or fourth rescuer):* Stabilize head end of long backboard.

Step 8: Secure patient to the backboard

- Crew carefully straps patient's torso first, head last, and then moves backboard to stretcher.
- Reassess PMS.

NOTE: *A wheeled stretcher can take the place of the fourth rescuer.*

➤ 55—RAPID TAKEDOWN OF STANDING PATIENT

Step 1: Rescuers get in position

- **Rescuer A:** Get in position behind patient and hold manual in-line stabilization of head and neck. Maintain manual stabilization until the patient is completely immobilized on a long backboard.
- **Rescuer B:** Get in position in front of patient. Explain procedure so patient does not move.

Step 2: Assess PMS and apply a cervical collar

- **Rescuer B:** Quickly assess pulses, motor ability, and sensory response (PMS) in all four extremities.
- **Rescuer B:** Apply a properly sized rigid extrication collar.

Step 3: Position the long backboard

- Position long backboard behind patient, being careful not to disturb manual stabilization in any way.
- Standing in front of patient to each side, reach under patient's armpit and grasp backboard handhold at level of armpit or higher. Both rescuers must hold same level.
- Then place your other hand on patient's upper arm, holding the patient against the backboard.

Step 4: Slowly lower the patient

- Slowly lower patient backwards, communicating with Rescuer A behind board so it is clear when the scapulae are beginning to rest on board. Remember to lift with your legs, bending at knees not at waist.

(continued)

Rescuer A gently allows the head to come back to board as shoulders come back.
- Once head is on board, it never is lifted off board again as Rescuer A kneels down at patient's head.
- Reassess PMS when the patient is finally down.

➤ 56—WATER RESCUE: POTENTIAL SPINE INJURY*

- Take BSI precautions and wear a personal floatation device (PFD).
- Conduct an initial assessment.
- Splint head and neck with arms. (Lift the patient's arms over his or her head. Then splint head and neck between arms.)
- Roll patient over into supine position.
- Assess airway and breathing.**
- Provide manual stabilization of head/neck.
- Assess pulses, motor ability, and sensory response (PMS) in four extremities.
- Slide backboard under patient.
- Apply a properly sized rigid extrication collar.
- Tie-down torso, then head/neck with straps.
- Float board to edge of the water.
- Remove patient from water with as much assistance as needed.
- Obtain baseline vital signs.
- Conduct focused history and physical exam.
- Reassess PMS in four extremities.
- Apply oxygen, and prepare to transport.

NOTES: * *MOI indicates high degree of head/neck injury.*
** *If patient is not breathing, begin ventilations and remove right away. If patient is in cardiac arrest, remove immediately as compressions are not done in the water.*

➤ 57—AIR MATTRESS

- Take BSI precautions.
- Direct assistant to place head in neutral, in-line position and to maintain manual stabilization until the patient is completely immobilized.
- Assess distal pulses, motor ability, and sensory response (PMS).
- Apply a properly sized rigid extrication collar.
- In order to carefully life the patient onto the air mattress, a scoop stretcher is recommended.
- Position the patient on the air mattress and remove the scoop stretcher.
- Evacuate the air from the mattress using the pump according to the manufacturer's instructions.
- Apply straps to the torso and the head.
- Reassess distal PMS.

➤ 58—ONE-RESCUER ASSIST

- Place patient's arm around your neck.
- Grasp patient's hand in your hand.
- Place your other arm around the patient's waist.
- Help patient walk to safety, communicating with him or her about obstacles or uneven terrain.

➤ 59—TWO-RESCUER ASSIST

- Each rescuer stands at one side of the patient.
- Each places a patient's arm around his or her shoulder and grips the patient's hand.
- Both rescuers then help the patient walk to safety.

➤ 60—EXTREMITY CARRY

Rescuer A:

- Place the patient on his or her back with knees flexed.
- Kneel at patient's head, and place your hands under patient's shoulders.

Rescuer B:

- Kneel at the patient's feet and grasp his or her wrists.
- Lift patient forward while Rescuer A slips arms under patient's armpits and grasps patient's wrists.
- Grasp patient's knees while facing patient, or turn and grasp patient's knees while facing away from patient.

Rescuers A and B:

- Crouch, then stand at the same time.
- Move as a unit when carrying the patient.

➤ 61—DIRECT CARRY

Rescuers A and B:

- Get in position along one side of patient. Rescuer A is at head-end; Rescuer B at foot-end.

Rescuer A:

- Cradle patient's head and neck by sliding one arm under patient's neck to grasp shoulder.

Rescuer B:

- Slide hand under patient's hip and lift slightly.

Rescuer A:

- Slide your other arm under patient's back.

Rescuer B:

- Place your arms under patient's hips and calves.

Rescuers A and B:

- Slide patient to edge of bed and bend toward him or her with your knees slightly bent.
- Then lift and curl patient to your chests and return to standing position.
- Rotate, and slide patient gently onto stretcher.

➤ 62—DIRECT GROUND LIFT

- Set stretcher in its lowest position, and place opposite patient.

Rescuers A and B:

- Get in position along one side of patient. Rescuer A is at head-end; Rescuer B at foot-end.

Rescuers A and B:

- Drop to one knee, facing patient.
- Then place patient's arms on his or her chest.

Rescuer A:

- Cradle patient's head and neck by sliding one arm under the neck to grasp shoulder; place your other arm under patient's lower back.

Rescuer B:

- Slide one arm under patient's knees and the other under patient above buttocks.
- If a third rescuer is available, he or she should place both arms under patient's waist while Rescuers A and B slide their arms up to mid-back or down to buttocks.
- On a signal, crew lifts patient to their knees.
- On a signal, crew members stand and carry patient to stretcher, drop to one knee, and roll forward to place patient onto mattress.

➤ 63—LOADING WHEELED STRETCHER

- Lift rear step of ambulance.
- Move stretcher as close to ambulance as possible.
- Make sure stretcher is locked in its lowest level before lifting (depends on local procedure and type of stretcher).

Rescuers A and B:

- Get in position on opposite sides of stretcher, bend at knees, and grasp lower bar of stretcher frame.
- Come to a full standing position with backs straight.
- Use oblique stepping movements to move stretcher to ambulance.
- Secure stretcher into ambulance using the appropriate securing device.
- Engage both forward and rear catches to hold stretcher in place.

➤ 64—CRADLE CARRY

- Place one arm across patient's back with your hand under his or her arm.

- Place your other arm under his or her knees and lift.

- If patient is conscious, have him or her place nearest arm over your shoulder.

➤ 65—FIREFIGHTER'S DRAG

- Place patient in supine position.
- Tie patient's hands together with something that will not cut into skin.
- Straddle patient, facing his or her head.
- Crouch and pass your head through patient's trussed arms, and then raise your body to raise patient's head, neck, and upper trunk.
- Crawl on your hands and knees, dragging patient and keeping patient's head low to ground.

➤ 66—BLANKET DRAG

- Gather half of blanket up against patient's side.
- Roll patient toward your knees.
- Gently roll patient onto blanket.
- Roll up blanket by patient's head, neck, and shoulders and drag this rolled material, keeping patient's head as low to ground as possible.

➤ 67—PACK STRAP CARRY

- Have patient stand.
- Turn your back to patient, bringing his or her arms over your shoulders to cross your chest.
- Keep patient's arms as straight as possible and armpits over your shoulders.
- Hold patient's wrists, bend, and pull patient onto your back.

➤ 68—PIGGYBACK CARRY

- Assist patient to a standing position.
- Turn your back to patient, placing patient's arms over your shoulders so the arms cross your chest.
- While patient holds on with his or her arms, crouch and grasp patient's thighs.
- Use a lifting motion to move patient onto your back.
- Pass your forearms under patient's knees and grasp his or her wrists.

➤ 69—FIREFIGHTER'S CARRY

- Place your toes against patient's toes, and pull patient toward you.
- Bend at waist and flex your knees.
- Duck and pull patient across your shoulder, keeping hold of one of his or her wrists.
- Use your free arm to reach between patient's legs and grasp thigh.
- Let weight of patient fall onto your shoulders.
- Stand up, transferring your grip on patient's thigh to his or her wrist.

➤ EFFECTS OF AGING

- *Depositing of cholesterol*—arterial walls become thicker, increasing the risk of heart attack, stroke, and hypertension.

- *Decreased cardiac output*—diminished activity and less tolerance of physical stress, making patient more prone to falls.

- *Decreased elasticity of lungs and decreased activity of cilia*—less ability to clear foreign substances from lungs, increasing risk of pneumonia.

- *Fewer taste buds, less saliva, less acid production, and slower movement in digestive system*—difficulty chewing and swallowing, less enjoyment of eating; difficulty digesting and absorbing food; increased constipation; early feeling of fullness when eating. These conditions make patient more prone to weight loss and abdominal pain.

- *Diminished liver and kidney function*—increased toxicity from alcohol and medications; diminished ability of blood to clot, which makes patient prone to bleed.

- *Decreased muscle mass and loss of minerals from bones*—decreased strength and increased risk for falls, leading to more fractures.

- *Multiple medical conditions*—high probability of many medications, sometimes prescribed by different physicians.

(continued)

- ***Death of friends and family***—increased risk of depression or loss of social support, which in turn increases the risk of suicide.

- ***Loss of skin elasticity and shrinking of sweat glands***—thin, dry, wrinkled skin, which increases risk of injury.

➤ MNEMONICS

SPLATT (adapted from JEMS, 2003, p. 105)

S—Symptoms.

P—Previous falls.

L—Location of fall.

A—Activity at time of fall.

T—Time of fall.

T—Trauma (physical or psychological).

VITAMINS CD (Origins of Mechanism for Nervous System Pathophysiology)

V—Vascular (stroke, brain, embolism).

I—Inflammation (of blood vessels of the brain).

T—Toxins (CO poisoning, trauma such as bleeding into the brain or concussion, tumors).

A—Autoimmune (immune system component production against CNS—MS and lupus).

M—Metabolic (liver or renal failure, hypo-/hyperglycemia, hypo-/hyperthyroidism).

I—Infection (meningitis, encephalitis).

N—Narcotics and other drugs causing mental status changes.

S—Systemic (sepsis, hypoxia).

C—Congenital (seizures).

D—Degenerative (Alzheimer disease and other dementias, Parkinson disease).

➤ 70—DEALING WITH PEDIATRIC PATIENTS

- Take BSI precautions.
- Identify yourself (simple/informal).
- Let child know someone will call parents.
- Determine if there are life-threatening problems and treat them immediately.
- Let child have a nearby toy.
- Kneel or sit at child's eye level.
- Make eye contact without staring.
- Smile.
- Touch child or hold his or her hand or foot if appropriate.
- Explain in simple terms equipment that you plan to use.
- Stop occasionally to confirm that child understands your actions.
- Never lie to a child.

➤ 71—CHILD SAFETY SEAT IMMOBILIZATION: ASSESSMENT

- Take BSI precautions.
- Then take the following steps.

Rescuer A:

- Get in position behind patient. Apply manual in-line stabilization of head and neck. Maintain manual stabilization throughout procedure.

- Based on initial assessment and patient's status, determine if he or she should be immobilized in seat (#72) or rapidly extricated (#73).

Rescuer B:

- Prepare equipment.

- Apply rigid extrication collar, or improvise a collar with rolled hand towel for newborn or infant.

- Place a small blanket or bath towel on child's lap. Either strap or use wide tape to secure pelvis and chest area to seat.

- Place a towel roll on both sides of head to fill voids. Tape forehead in place. Then place tape across collar or maxilla. Avoid taping chin, which would place pressure on child's neck and close airway.

- Carry patient and seat to ambulance and strap them onto stretcher with stretcher head raised.

- Reassess distal PMS.

➤ 72—IMMOBILIZING PATIENT IN A CHILD SAFETY SEAT

- Take BSI precautions.
- Then follow these steps.

Rescuer A:

- Stabilize child safety seat in an upright position.
- Maintain manual stabilization of head and neck throughout procedure until patient is completely immobilized.

Rescuer B:

- Prepare equipment.
- Apply rigid extrication collar, or improvise a collar with rolled hand towel for newborn or infant.
- Place a small blanket or bath towel on child's lap. Either strap or use wide tape to secure pelvis and chest area to seat.
- Place a towel roll on both sides of head to fill voids. Tape forehead in place. Then place tape across collar or maxilla. Avoid taping chin, which would place pressure on child's neck and close airway.
- Carry patient and seat to ambulance.
- Strap them onto stretcher with stretcher head raised.
- Reassess PMS.

➤ 73—CHILD SAFETY SEAT: RAPID EXTRICATION

- Take BSI precautions.
- Then follow these steps.

Rescuer A:

- Stabilize child safety seat in upright position.
- Maintain manual stabilization of head and neck throughout procedure until patient is completely immobilized.

Rescuer B:

- Prepare equipment.
- Loosen or cut car seat straps and false front guard.
- Apply rigid extrication collar, or improvise with rolled hand towel in newborn/infant.
- Place child safety seat on center of long backboard and slowly tilt it back into a supine position, being careful not to allow patient to slide out of chair. If patient has a large head, it is helpful to place a towel under area where shoulders will end up on board.

Rescuer A:

- Call for a coordinated long axis move onto board.
- Continue to maintain manual stabilization of head and neck.

Rescuer B:

- Grasp chest and axilla with each hand and do a coordinated long axis move onto board. Make sure

(continued)

child is positioned at the end of the board and not in the middle.

- Place a rolled blanket on each side of patient.
- Strap pelvis and upper chest to board. Do not strap abdomen down. Tape lower legs to board with wide tape.
- Place a towel roll on both sides of head to fill voids. Tape forehead in place. Then place tape across collar or maxilla. Do not tape across chin to avoid pressure on patient's neck.
- Reassess PMS.

NOTE: *Make sure the seat is not damaged.*

➤ CHARACTERISTICS OF ANATOMY AND PHYSIOLOGY

- Tongue is proportionately larger than an adult's and more likely to block the airway.
- Smaller airway is more easily blocked.
- Abundant secretions can block the airway.
- Baby teeth are easily broken and can block the airway.
- Flat nose and face is hard to get a good mask seal.
- Big head and weak neck muscles are prone to trauma.
- Open fontanelles may indicate rising intracranial pressure (ICP) if bulging or dehydration if sunken.
- Short narrow trachea can close easily with hyperextension of the neck.
- Short neck is difficult to immobilize.
- Children tend to be abdominal breathers.
- Prolonged periods of rapid respiratory rate cause tiring and ultimately lead to respiratory distress.
- Larger body surface area (BSA) makes the patient prone to hypothermia.
- Thinner skin is more sensitive to burns.
- Softer bones are more flexible, which when injured result in fewer fractures and more internal damage.
- Spleen and liver are more exposed, which makes them more prone to injury.
- Infants are primarily nose breathers.

➤ DEVELOPMENTAL CHARACTERISTICS

Newborns and Infants—Birth to 1 Year

- Do not like to be separated from parents.
- Minimal stranger anxiety.
- Used to being undressed, but like to feel warm.
- Follow movements with eyes.
- Do not want to be "suffocated" by oxygen mask.

Toddlers—1 to 3 Years

- Do not like to be touched or separated from parents.
- Believe their illness is a punishment for being bad.
- Do not like having clothing removed.
- Frighten easily and overreact.
- Have begun to assert independence.
- Do not want to be "suffocated" by oxygen mask.

Preschool—3 to 5 Years

- Do not like to be touched or separated from parents.
- Modest and do not like clothing removed.
- Believe that their illness is a punishment for being bad.
- Fear of blood, pain, and permanent injury.
- Curious, communicative, and can be cooperative.
- Do not want to be "suffocated" by an oxygen mask.

(continued)

School Age—6 to 10 Years

- Cooperative but like opinions heard.
- Fear blood, pain, disfigurement, and permanent injury.
- Modest and do not like their bodies exposed.

Adolescents—11 to 18 Years

- Want to be treated as adults.
- Feel they are indestructible but may have fears of permanent injury and disfigurement.
- Vary in emotional and physical development and may not be comfortable with their changing bodies.

NOTE: *For purposes of resuscitation by health care providers, a child is from 1 year to the age of developing secondary sexual charistics (puberty).*

➤ ADDITIONAL SIGNIFICANT MOI FOR A CHILD

- Falls from more than 10 feet.
- Bicycle collision.
- Vehicle in medium-speed collision.

➤ **STAGES OF LABOR**

First stage:
beginning of contractions
to full cervical dilation

Second stage:
baby enters birth canal and is born

Third stage:
delivery of the placenta

➤ 74—ASSESSMENT OF MOTHER FOR IMMINENT DELIVERY

- Take BSI precautions.
- Conduct an initial assessment.
- Obtain mother's history to determine active labor. History includes:
  - Length of term.
  - Number of previous pregnancies and births.
  - Frequency and duration of uterine contractions.
  - Recent vaginal discharge or hemorrhage.
  - Whether or not "water broke" yet.
  - Presence of strain or urge to move bowels.
- With mother's permission, examine for crowning.
- Feel for uterine contractions when mother says she is having one.
- Take a set of vitals and make decision: prepare for delivery or begin transport.

➤ **NEWBORN RESUSCITATION**

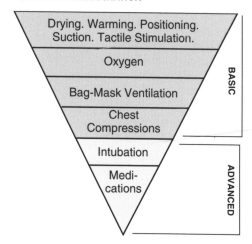

➤ APGAR SCORE

		Points	Score	
			1 min	5 min
A	APPEARANCE (SKIN COLOR)			
	Blue or pale extremities	0		
	Pink trunk and blue extremities	1		
	Completely pink	2	_____	_____
P	PULSE			
	Absent	0		
	<100	1		
	>100	2	_____	_____
G	GRIMACE (IRRITABILITY)			
	No response	0		
	Grimace or whimpers	1		
	Actively cries	2	_____	_____
A	ACTIVITY (MUSCLE TONE)			
	Flaccid, limp	0		
	Some flexion of extremities	1		
	Active extremity motion	2	_____	_____
R	RESPIRATORY EFFORT			
	Absent	0		
	Slow and irregular	1		
	Strong cry	2	_____	_____
	TOTAL SCORE		_____	

(continued)

Ideally, scores are taken at 1 and 5 minutes after birth. If the neonate is not breathing, DO NOT withhold resuscitation for an APGAR score. Total scores indicate the following:

7–10   indicates an active and vigorous neonate who requires routine care.

4–6   indicates a moderately depressed neonate who requires oxygenation and stimulation.

0–3   indicates a severely depressed neonate who requires immediate resuscitation.

By assessing the APGAR score at 1 minute and repeating at 5 minutes, it is possible to determine whether or not intervention has caused a change in the newlyborn's status.

➤ 75—MANAGEMENT OF ABSORBED POISONS

- Size up situation, and take the necessary precautions to prevent injury to yourself and your crew.

- Remove patient from source. Avoid contaminating yourself with poison.

- Conduct an initial assessment.

- Maintain an open airway.

- Administer high-concentration oxygen.

- Perform a focused history and physical exam, including SAMPLE history and vital signs.

- Brush powders from patient. Be careful not to abrade patient's skin.

- Remove contaminated clothing and other articles, such as shoes and jewelry.

- Quickly gather information about product.

- If appropriate, irrigate with large amounts of clear water for at least 20 minutes. Call medical direction.

- Perform ongoing assessment.

- Be alert for shock, and transport as soon as possible.

➤ 76—MANAGEMENT OF INGESTED POISONS (EMT-B SKILL)

- Take BSI precautions.
- Conduct an initial assessment.
- Maintain an open airway.
- Perform a focused history and physical exam, including SAMPLE history and vital signs.
- Quickly gather information about substance.
- Call medical direction on scene or en route.
- If directed, administer activated charcoal.
- Position patient for vomiting and save all vomitus. Have suction ready.
- Perform ongoing assessment.
- Transport as soon as possible.

➤ 77—MANAGEMENT OF INHALED POISONS

- Size up the situation, and take the necessary precautions to prevent injury to yourself and your crew.*

- Remove patient from the source. Avoid contaminating yourself with poison.

- Maintain open airway. Stay alert for vomiting. Properly position the patient and have suction equipment ready.

- Conduct an initial assessment.

- Administer high-concentration oxygen by nonrebreather mask.

- Perform a focused history and physical exam, including a SAMPLE history.

- Remove contaminated clothing and other articles (e.g., shoes, jewelry).

- Assess baseline vital signs.

- Quickly gather information about product (e.g., containers, bottles, and labels).

- Call medical direction on scene or en route.

- Transport as soon as possible.

- Perform ongoing assessment en route.

SAFETY NOTE: In the presence of hazardous fumes or gases, wait for those who are properly trained and equipped to enter scene and remove patient to a safe area.

➤ CLASSIFICATION OF BURNS BY DEPTH

Superficial | Partial thickness | Full thickness

Skin reddened | Blisters | Charring

Epidermis
Dermis
Fat
Muscle

➤ RULE OF NINES—ADULTS

Adult

9%

9%

4 1/2%   4 1/2%

9%   9%

9%

9%

1%

4 1/2%

9%   9%

9%   9%

➤ RULE OF NINES—INFANTS AND CHILDREN

Child

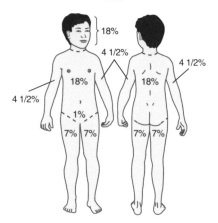

18%

4 1/2%

18%

4 1/2%

4 1/2%

18%

1%

7% 7%

7% 7%

Infant

14%   9%

1%   18%

14%   9%

Front 18%
Back 18%

➤ CLASSIFICATION OF BURN SEVERITY

Minor Burns—Adults

- Full-thickness burns <2 percent of body surface, excluding face, hands, feet, genitalia, or respiratory tract.
- Partial-thickness burns <15 percent of body surface.
- Superficial burns ≤50 percent of body surface.

Minor Burns—Children <5 Years Old

- Partial-thickness burns <10 percent of body surface.

Moderate Burns—Adults

- Full-thickness burns of 2–10 percent of body surface, excluding face, hands, feet, genitalia, or respiratory tract.
- Partial-thickness burns of 15–30 percent of body surface.
- Superficial burns that involve more than 50 percent of body surface.

Moderate Burns—Children <5 Years Old

- Partial-thickness burns of 10–20 percent of body surface.

Critical Burns—Adults

- All burns complicated by injuries of respiratory tract, other soft-tissue injuries, and bone injuries.
- Partial- or full-thickness burns of face, feet, hands, genitalia, or respiratory tract.
- Full-thickness burns >10 percent of body surface.

(continued)

- Partial-thickness burns >30 percent of body surface.
- Burns complicated by musculoskeletal injuries.
- Circumferential burns.

Critical Burns—Children < 5 Years Old

- Full-thickness or partial-thickness burns
  > 20 percent of body surface.

➤ 78—ACTIVE RAPID REWARMING OF FROZEN PARTS

- Take BSI precautions.
- Conduct an initial assessment.
- Conduct focused history and physical exam, including taking baseline vital signs.
- Consider administering oxygen by nonrebreather mask.
- Heat water to a temperature between 100°F and 105°F.
- Fill container with heated water and prepare injured part by removing clothing, jewelry, bands, or straps.
- Fully immerse injured part. Do not allow injured area to touch sides or bottom of container. Do not place any pressure on affected part. Continuously stir the water. When water cools below 100°F, remove affected part and add more warm water. The patient may complain of moderate pain as the affected area rewarms or may experience periods of intense pain.
- If you complete rewarming of the part, gently dry the affected area and apply a dry sterile dressing.
- Place dry sterile dressings between fingers and toes before dressing hands/feet.
- Cover the site with blankets or whatever is available to keep affected area warm. Do not allow these coverings to come in contact with injured area or to put pressure on site.
- Keep patient at rest. Do not allow patient to walk if a lower extremity has been frostbitten or frozen.
- Keep entire patient warm.

(continued)

- Continue to monitor the patient.

- Assist circulation according to local protocol. (Some systems recommend rhythmically and carefully raising and lowering affected limb.)

- Do not allow limb to refreeze.

- Transport patient as soon as possible, with affected limb slightly elevated.

Signs and symptoms of hypothermia.

WIND SPEED (MPH)	WHAT THE THERMOMETER READS (degrees °F.)											
	50	40	30	20	10	0	−10	−20	−30	−40	−50	−60
CALM	WHAT IT EQUALS IN ITS EFFECT ON EXPOSED FLESH											
CALM	50	40	30	20	10	0	−10	−20	−30	−40	−50	−60
5	48	37	27	16	6	−5	−15	−26	−36	−47	−57	−68
10	40	28	16	4	−9	−21	−33	−46	−58	−70	−83	−95
15	36	22	9	−5	−18	−36	−45	−58	−72	−85	−99	−112
20	32	18	4	−10	−25	−39	−53	−67	−82	−96	−110	−121
25	30	16	0	−15	−29	−44	−59	−74	−88	−104	−118	−133
30	28	13	−2	−18	−33	−48	−63	−79	−94	−109	−125	−140
35	27	11	−4	−20	−35	−49	−67	−82	−98	−113	−129	−145
40	26	10	−6	−21	−37	−53	−69	−85	−100	−116	−132	−148
	Little danger if properly clothed				Danger of freezing exposed flesh				Great danger of freezing exposed flesh			

Source: U.S. Army

Wind-chill index.

➤ 79—PATIENT REFUSAL PROCEDURE

- Spend time effectively communicating with patient (includes reasoning, persistence, and strategies to convince patient to go to hospital).

- Clearly inform patient of consequences of not going to hospital.

- Consult with medical direction.

- Contact family to help convince patient.

- Call law enforcement who may be able to order or "arrest" serious patient in order to force patient to go to hospital.

- Try to determine why patient is refusing care.

- Complete thorough documentation of refusal, have patient sign refusal release, and have witness sign the release (e.g., bystander, police, family).

NOTE: *Procedure may differ by state and jurisdiction. Always follow your medical director's advice.*

➤ 80–HANDWASHING/USE OF PPE

- Remove watch and rings. Roll up sleeves.
- Adjust water flow and temperature.
- Wet hands and distal forearms.
- Dispense soap onto hands.
- Scrub lower arms and hands. Clean around and under nails.
- Rinse thoroughly under running water to remove all soap. Do not touch sink!
- Use a paper towel to shut off faucet in order to avoid recontamination of hands.

Even though the EMS provider wears protective gloves with all patients, handwashing must still be performed immediately after each call.

(*continued*)

PPE CONSIDERATIONS

Equipment/Supply Item	Recommended Use
Latex-free disposable gloves	All patient contacts that could involve body substances (blood, urine, secretions, etc.). Cleaning the suction unit or cleaning up blood spills.
Eye shield or goggles	All patient contacts involving airway management, spurting blood, emergency childbirth, or a patient with a cough.
Standard surgical mask	All patient contacts involving airway management, spurting blood, emergency childbirth, or a patient with a cough.
HEPA, N-95, or NIOSH approved mask	Any patient with a potential for active Tb.
Helmet and goggles	Any rescue scene.
Heavy coat and pants	Any rescue scene.
Leather (gardening style) gloves	Any rescue scene.

➤ 81—TRANSFERRING THE PATIENT

• Take BSI precautions.

• Transfer patient as soon as possible. In a routine admission or when an illness or injury is not life-threatening, first check to see what is to be done with patient.

• A rescuer should remain with patient until transfer is complete.

• Assist emergency department staff as required.

• Give a complete verbal report of patient's condition and treatment administered.

• Complete your prehospital care report (PCR) and turn a copy over to hospital staff.

• Transfer patient's personal effects.

• Obtain your release from hospital if required in your region.

➤ 82—ACTIONS TO BE TAKEN AT HOSPITAL

- Take BSI precautions.
- Clean ambulance interior as required by your service exposure control plan.
- Replace respiratory equipment as required.
- Replace disposable items according to local policies.
- Exchange equipment according to local policies.
- Make up ambulance stretcher.

➤ 83—TERMINATION OF ACTIVITIES IN QUARTERS

- Place contaminated linens in biohazard container and noncontaminated linens in regular hamper.

- Remove and clean patient care equipment as required.

- Clean and sanitize respiratory equipment as needed.

- Clean and sanitize ambulance interior as required. Use germicide on devices and surfaces that were in contact with blood and body fluids.

- Wash thoroughly and change soiled clothing.

- Replace expendable supplies and equipment as required.

NOTE: Be sure to follow your agency's exposure control plan for cleaning and disinfecting procedures.

➤ 84—CLEANING AND DISINFECTING EQUIPMENT

- Use *low-level disinfectant*—one approved by the EPA, such as Lysol®, to clean and kill germs on ambulance floors and walls.

- Use *intermediate-level disinfectant*—such as a mixture of 1:100 bleach-to-water to clean and kill germs on equipment.

- Use *high-level disinfectant*—such as Cidex Plus®, to destroy all forms of microbial life except high numbers of bacterial spores.

NOTE: *Sterilization is required to destroy all possible sources of infection on equipment that will be used invasively.*

➤ DANGEROUS AREAS NEAR A HELICOPTER

➤ 85—ESTABLISHING COMMAND AT A MULTIPLE-CASUALTY INCIDENT (MCI)

- Perform a scene size-up.
- Locate police and fire officers and establish a unified command post.
- Don EMS command vest.
- Notify EMS dispatcher:
  - Designate EMS operations officer (as ruled).
  - Declare an MCI.
  - Indicate extent of incident.
  - Note whether ongoing or contained.
  - Estimate number of patients.
  - Identify location of command post.
  - Request number of BLS/ALS units.
- Designate a triage officer.
- Designate a staging officer:
  - Select location for staging sector.
  - Notify dispatcher to have all additional ambulances respond to staging.
- Request dispatcher roll call hospitals for bed availability.
- Designate treatment officer and location for this sector (as needed).

(continued)

- Designate transportation officer and location for this sector (as needed).
  - Consider need for aeromedical evacuation and appropriate landing zone near scene.
  - Consider usefulness of a school bus to transport walking wounded (low-priority) patients. Make sure everyone on bus is medically examined and that medical personnel also ride bus.
- Consider need for extrication sector (if not already established).
- Consider need for a safety officer (as needed).
- Consider need for rehab of personnel.
- Keep dispatcher and other service chiefs in close contact throughout incident.
- Along with police and fire officers, consider need for a public information officer to work with arriving media.

Special Operations

➤ MCI TERMS AND DEFINITIONS

EMS Operations—the person who is responsible for the actual operations of the incident.

IMS—incident management system.

Jump START—the pediatric triage plan.

MCI—multiple-casualty incident.

NIMS—national incident management system.

Rehab Sector—the location where emergency service providers are sent to be rehydrated, cooled off, and to obtain rest and medical monitoring of vital signs if needed.

Safety Officer—the person assigned at large-scale incidents to ensure safety of all EMS personnel at the scene.

Singular Command—single agency controls all resources and operations at an MCI.

Staging Sector—the dedicated area where resources including personnel, vehicles, and equipment are held until needed on scene.

START—simple triage and rapid transport.

Transport Sector—an area established for ambulance loading and supervised patient evacuation. The destinations of all patients are logged here.

Treatment Sector—a designated area set up to treat patients prior to transport.

Triage Sector—an area established for reassessment and removal of patients for a treatment sector.

(continued)

Triage—sorting or setting priorities for patient treatment.

Unified Command—the commanding officers from each public safety agency working together to make key decisions at an MCI.

➤ PATIENT TRIAGE PRIORITIES

P–1—Treatable life-threatening illness or injuries, including airway and breathing difficulties, uncontrolled or severe bleeding, decreased mental status, patients with severe medical problems, shock, severe burns. (Red-colored designation)

P–2—Serious but not life-threatening illness or injuries including burns without airway problems, major or multiple bone or joint injuries, back injuries with or without spinal-cord damage. (Yellow-colored designation)

P–3—"Walking wounded" including minor musculoskeletal injuries, minor soft-tissue injuries. (Green-colored designation)

P–4—*(sometimes called Priority 0):* Dead or fatally injured, including exposed brain matter, cardiac arrest (no pulse for more than 20 minutes, except with cold-water drowning or severe hypothermia), decapitation, severed trunk, and incineration. (Black-colored designation)

➤ 86–START TRIAGE

START stands for simple triage and rapid treatment. It relies on a simple approach to take no longer than 30 seconds per patient.

The physiologic parameters can be remembered with the acronym RPM (respirations, pulse, mental status).

Begin by asking those patients who can walk to get up and move to a nearby collection point. These patients are walking wounded or green tags (Priority 3).

(continued)

Now focus your attention on those patients who are unable to walk, hear, or follow commands using the chart below:

START Triage

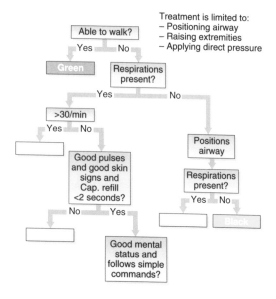

➤ 87–JUMPSTART PEDIATRIC MCI TRIAGE

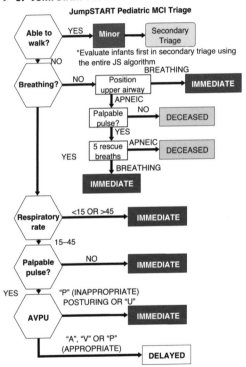

The JumpSTART pediatric MCI triage system.
(Copyright 2002 Lou E. Romig, MD, FAAP, FACEP)

➤ **WEAPONS OF MASS DESTRUCTION: SIGNS AND SYMPTOMS OF EXPOSURE TO A NERVE AGENT**

Remember the acronym (SLUDGEM-Resp-Agitation):

- **S**alivation or excessive drooling
- **L**acrimation or tearing
- **U**rination
- **D**efecation or diarrhea
- **G**astrointestinal upset (cramps)
- **E**mesis or vomiting
- **M**uscle twitching or spasm
- **R**espiration—difficulty breathing and wheezing
- **A**gitation + CNS signs of confusion, agitation, seizures, or coma

➤ WEAPONS OF MASS DESTRUCTION: RECOGNIZE HARM POSED BY THREAT

Remember the acronym TRACEM-P

Thermal—caused by extreme heat.

Radiological—danger from alpha or beta particles, or gamma rays (see figure below).

Asphyxiation—a lack of oxygen in the atmosphere.

Chemical—toxic or corrosive materials (e.g., sulfuric acid, lye, cyanide, nerve agents).

Etiological—disease-causing organisms (e.g., bacteria, viruses, or other toxins).

Mechanical—bombs and detonations.

Psychological—spreading fear.

The relative penetrating power of alpha, beta, and gamma radiation.

➤ HAZMAT CLASSIFICATION SYSTEM

United Nations HazMat Classification System	Placards Found in Transit
Class 1: Explosives	
Division 1.1	Explosives with a mass explosive hazard
Division 1.2	Explosives with a projection hazard
Division 1.3	Explosives with predominantly a fire hazard
Division 1.4	Explosives with no significant blast hazard
Division 1.5	Very insensitive explosives or blasting agents
Division 1.6	Extremely insensitive detonating articles
Class 2: Gases	
Division 2.1	Flammable gases
Division 2.2	Nonflammable, nontoxic, compressed gases
Division 2.3	Gases toxic by inhalation
Division 2.4	Corrosive gases
Class 3: Flammable Liquids and Combustible Liquids	

(continued)

United Nations HazMat Classification System	Placards Found in Transit

Class 4: Flammable Solids

Division 4.1	Flammable solids
Division 4.2	Spontaneously combustible materials
Division 4.3	Dangerous-when-wet materials

Class 5: Oxidizers and Organic Peroxides

Division 5.1	Oxidizers
Division 5.2	Organic peroxides

Class 6: Toxic Materials and Infectious Substances

Division 6.1	Toxic materials
Division 6.2	Infectious substances

Class 7: Radioactive Materials

Class 8: Corrosive Materials

Class 9: Miscellaneous Dangerous Goods

Division 9.1	Miscellaneous dangerous goods
Division 9.2	Environmentally hazardous substances
Division 9.3	Dangerous wastes

➤ MUSCULOSKELETAL SYSTEM

Skull (Cranium)
Orbit (Eye Socket)
Zygomatic Bone
Cervical Vertebra (Neck)
Sternum (Breast Bone)
Xiphoid Process
Costal Cartilage
Lumbar Vertebra
Illiac Crest
Ilium (Hip)
Pelvic Girdle
Greater Trochanter
Lesser Trochanter
Symphysis Pubis

Frontal
Parietal
Occipital
Temporal
Temporomandibular Joint
Maxilla
Mandible
Acromioclavicular Joint
Glenohumeral Joint
Scapula (Shoulder Blade)
Ribs
Humerus (Arm Bone)
Elbow
Forearm
Ulna
Radius
Sacrum

Clavicle (Collarbone)

Ischium
Coccyx (Tail Bone)
Carpals (Wrist)
Metacarpals (Hand)
Phalanges (Fingers)
Femur (Thigh Bone)
Patella (Knee Cap)

Lower Leg Bones

Tibia
Fibula

Tarsals (Ankle)
Metatarsals (Foot)
Phalanges (Toes)
Calcaneus (Heel)

➤ NERVOUS SYSTEM

The Brain

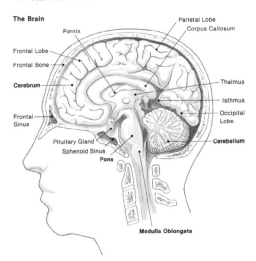

Fornix

Parietal Lobe
Corpus Callosum

Frontal Lobe

Frontal Bone

Cerebrum

Thalamus

Isthmus

Occipital Lobe

Frontal Sinus

Pituitary Gland

Sphenoid Sinus

Cerebellum

Pons

Medulla Oblongata

➤ DIVISIONS OF THE SPINAL CORD

Divisions of the
Spinal Cord

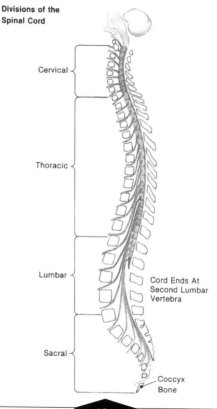

Cervical

Thoracic

Lumbar

Cord Ends At
Second Lumbar
Vertebra

Sacral

Coccyx
Bone

➤ CRANIAL HEMATOMAS

Dura

Dura

Subdural

Epidural

Intracerebral

➤ DIGESTIVE SYSTEM

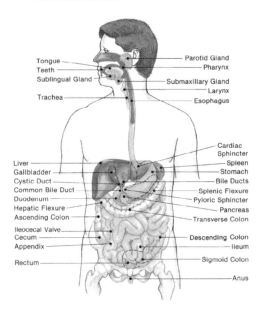

Tongue
Teeth
Sublingual Gland
Trachea

Parotid Gland
Pharynx
Submaxillary Gland
Larynx
Esophagus

Cardiac Sphincter
Spleen
Stomach
Bile Ducts
Splenic Flexure
Pyloric Sphincter
Pancreas
Transverse Colon

Liver
Gallbladder
Cystic Duct
Common Bile Duct
Duodenum
Hepatic Flexure
Ascending Colon
Ileocecal Valve
Cecum
Appendix
Rectum

Descending Colon
Ileum
Sigmoid Colon
Anus

➤ URINARY SYSTEM

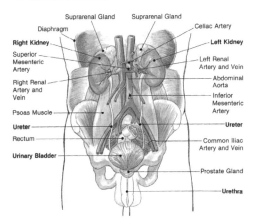

➤ RELATED TERMS

Indications—specific signs, symptoms, or circumstances under which it is appropriate to administer a drug to a patient.

Contraindications—specific signs, symptoms, or circumstances under which it is not appropriate, and may be harmful, to administer a drug to a patient.

Side Effect—any action of a drug other than the desired action.

➤ DRUG ADMINISTRATION PROCEDURE

Before administering a drug:

1. Confirm the order.
2. Write it down.
3. Check "five rights":
   - Do I have the right patient?
   - Is this the right medication?
   - Is this the right dose?
   - Is this the right time for the medication to be given?
   - Am I giving this medication by the right route of administration?

➤ ACTIVATED CHARCOAL

Medication Name

- Generic: activated charcoal.

- Trade: SuperChar®, InstaChar®, Actidose®, Liqui-Char®, and others.

Indications

- Poisoning by mouth.

Contraindications

- Altered mental status.

- Ingestion of acids or alkalis.

- Inability to swallow.

Medication Form

- Premixed in water, frequently available in plastic bottle containing 12.5g of activated charcoal.

- Powder should be avoided in field.

Dosage

- Adults and children: 1g activated charcoal/kg of body weight.

- Usual adult dose: 25–50 g.

- Usual pediatric dose: 12.5–25 g.

Administration

- Consult medical direction/or poison control center.

- Shake container thoroughly.

- Because medication looks like mud, patient may need to be persuaded to drink it. Providing a covered

(continued)

container and a straw will prevent patient from
seeing the medication and so may improve patient
compliance.

- If patient does not drink the medication right away,
the charcoal will settle. Shake or stir it again before
administering.

- Record the name, dose, route, and time of
administration of the medication.

Actions

- Activated charcoal absorbs (binds) certain poisons
and prevents them from being absorbed into the body.

- Not all brands of activated charcoal are the same:
some absorb much more than others, so consult
medical direction about the brand to use.

Side Effects

- Black stools.

- Some patients, particularly those who have ingested
poisons that cause nausea, may vomit. If patient
vomits, repeat the dose once.

Reassessment Strategies

- Be prepared for the patient to vomit or to deteriorate
further.

POISON Help®

1-800-222-1222

The American Association of Poison Control
Center number redirects the caller to the
closest or most appropriate poison control
center.

➤ EPINEPHRINE AUTO-INJECTOR

Medication Name

- Generic: epinephrine.
- Trade: Adrenalin.
- Delivery system: EpiPen® or EpiPen® Jr.

Indications

Must meet the following three criteria:

- Patient exhibits signs of a severe allergic reaction, including either respiratory distress or shock.
- Medication is prescribed for this patient by a physician.
- Medical direction authorizes use for this patient.

Contraindications

- No contraindications when used in a life-threatening situation.

Medication Form

- Liquid administered by an auto-injector (an automatically injectable needle-and-syringe system).

Dosage

- Adults: one adult auto-injector (0.3 mg).
- Infant and child: one infant/child auto-injector (0.15 mg).

Administration

- Obtain patient's prescribed auto-injector. Ensure prescription is written for the patient who is experiencing the severe allergic reaction. Ensure medication is not discolored (if visible).

(continued)

173

- Obtain order from medical direction, either on-line or off-line.
- Remove cap from auto-injector. Place tip of auto-injector against patient's thigh (lateral portion, midway between waist and knee).
- Push the injector firmly against the thigh until the injector activates.
- Hold the injector in place until the medication is injected (at least 10 seconds).
- Record activity and time.
- Dispose of injector in biohazard container.

Actions

- Dilates the bronchioles.
- Constricts blood vessels.

Side Effects

- Increased heart rate.
- Pallor.
- Dizziness.
- Chest pain.
- Headache.
- Nausea, vomiting.
- Excitability, anxiety.

(continued)

Reassessment Strategies

- Transport.
- Continue focused assessment of airway, breathing, and circulatory status.
- If patient's condition continues to worsen (decreasing mental status, increased breathing difficulty, decreasing blood pressure):
  - Obtain medical direction for an additional dose of epinephrine.
  - Treat for shock.
  - Prepare to initiate basic life-support procedures (CPR, AED).
- If patient's condition improves, provide supportive care. That is, continue oxygen and treat for shock.

➤ NITROGLYCERIN

Medication Name

- Generic: nitroglycerin.
- Trade: Nitrostat®, Nitrolingual Spray®.

Indications

All of the following conditions must be met:

- Patient complains of chest pain.
- Patient with history of cardiac problems.
- Patient's physician has prescribed nitroglycerin (NTG).
- Systolic blood pressure is greater than 100.
- Medical direction authorizes administration of the medication.

Contraindications

- Patient has hypotension or a systolic blood pressure below 90 (or <30 mmHg below baseline).
- Patient has a head injury.
- Patient is an infant or child.
- Patient has already taken the maximum prescribed dose.
- Bradycardia <50 or tachycardia >100.
- Do not administer within 24 hours of Viagra (sildenafilcitrate) and Levitra (vardenafil) or within 48 hours of Cialis (tadalafil) administration (erectile dysfunction meds).

Medication Form

- Tablet, sublingual spray.

(continued)

Dosage

- One dose, repeat in 5 minutes. If no relief, if systolic blood pressure remains above 100, and if authorized by medical direction, up to a maximum of three doses.

Administration

- Perform focused assessment for cardiac patient.
- Take blood pressure. (Systolic pressure must be above 100.)
- Contact medical direction if no standing orders.
- Assure right medication, right patient, right dose, right route, right time.
- Check expiration date.
- Assure patient is alert.
- Question patient on last dose taken and effects.
- Assure understanding of route of administration.
- Ask patient to lift tongue. Place tablet under it (while wearing gloves), or spray on or under tongue.
- Have patient keep mouth closed with tablet under tongue (without swallowing) until dissolved and absorbed.
- Recheck blood pressure within 2 minutes.
- Record administration, route, and time.
- Perform reassessment.

Actions

- Relaxes blood vessels.
- Decreases workload of heart.

(continued)

Side Effects
- Hypotension (lowers blood pressure).
- Headache.
- Pulse rate changes.

Reassessment Strategies
- Monitor blood pressure.
- Ask patient about effect on pain relief.
- Seek medical direction before readministration.
- Record assessments.

➤ ORAL GLUCOSE

Medication Name

- Generic: Glucose, oral.
- Trade: Glutose®, Insta-glucose®.

Indications

- Altered mental status with a known history of diabetes mellitus.

Contraindications

- Unresponsiveness.
- Known diabetic has not taken insulin for days.
- Inability to swallow.

Medication Form

- Gel, in toothpaste-type tubes.

Dosage

- One tube.

Administration

- Assure signs and symptoms of altered mental status with a known history of diabetes.
- Assure patient is awake with a gag reflex.
- Administer glucose:
  - Place on tongue depressor between cheek and gum.
  - Self-administered between cheek and gum.
  - Perform ongoing assessment.

(continued)

Actions

- Increases blood sugar.

Side Effects

- None when given properly. May be aspirated by the patient without a gag reflex.

Reassessment Strategies

- If patient loses consciousness or seizes, remove tongue depressor from mouth.

➤ PRESCRIBED INHALER

Medication Name

- Generic: albuterol, isoetharine, metaproterenol.
- Trade: Proventil®, Ventolin®, Bronkosol®, Bronkometer®, Alupent®, Metaprel®.

Indications

Meets all of the following criteria:

- Patient exhibits signs and symptoms of respiratory emergency.
- Patient has physician-prescribed, hand-held inhaler.
- Medical direction gives specific authorization to use.

Contraindications

- Patient is unable to use device (e.g., not alert).
- Inhaler is not prescribed for patient.
- No permission has been given by medical direction.
- Patient has already taken maximum prescribed dose prior to EMT-B's arrival.

Medication Form

- Hand-held metered dose inhaler.

Dosage

- Number of inhalations based on medical director's order or physician's order.

Administration

- Obtain order from medical direction, either on-line or off-line.

(continued)

- Assure right patient, right medication, right dose, right route, right time, and patient alert enough to use inhaler.
- Check expiration date of inhaler.
- Check if patient has already taken any doses.
- Assure inhaler is at room temperature or warmer.
- Shake inhaler vigorously several times.
- Have patient exhale deeply.
- Have patient put lips around opening of inhaler.
- Have patient depress the hand-held inhaler as he or she begins to inhale deeply.
- Instruct patient to hold breath for as long as comfortable so medication can be absorbed.
- Put oxygen back on patient.
- Allow patient to breathe a few times, and repeat second dose if so ordered by medical direction.
- If patient has a spacer device for inhaler, it should be used.

Actions

- Beta agonist bronchodilator dilates bronchioles, reducing airway resistance.

Side Effects

- Increased pulse rate.
- Tremors.
- Nervousness.

(continued)

Reassessment Strategies

- Gather vital signs.
- Perform focused reassessment of chest and respiratory function.
- Observe for deterioration of patient; if breathing becomes inadequate, provide artificial respirations.

➤ CHEWABLE ASPIRIN

According to the AHA Guidelines 2005, "To improve Acute Coronary Syndrome (ACS) outcome, all dispatchers and EMS providers must be trained to recognize its symptoms. EMS providers should be trained to determine onset of ACS symptoms, stabilize the patient, and provide pre-arrival notification and transport to an appropriate medical care facility. EMS providers can support the airway, administer oxygen guided by oxygen saturation monitoring as available (*Class 11b*), and administer aspirin and nitroglycerin."

"If the patient has not taken aspirin and has no history of aspirin allergy, EMS providers should give the patient (162 to 325 mg) aspirin to chew (*Class 1*) and notify the receiving hospital before arrival."

Locally, this administration of aspirin and nitro requires authorization of medical direction. Your EMS system may have a standing order in place for this situation. *Check with your service medical director to see what the local policy is.*

The medications listed in this section are commonly used by patients. Generic names are lowercase; trade names are capitalized and in boldface type.

The class of each medication is listed. These classes are described as follows; a list of "meds" follows.

➤ CLASSES OF MEDICATIONS

ACE inhibitor—relaxes arteries and promotes renal excretion of salt and water.

Acid/peptic—controls excessive acid in the stomach.

Analgesic—relieves pain.

Anorexiant—reduces appetite.

Antianginal—prevents or relieves angina pectoris.

Antianxiety—prevents or reduces anxiety.

Antiarrhythmic—counteracts or prevents cardiac dysrhythmias.

Antiasthmatic—relieves the symptoms of asthma.

Antibiotic—helps destroy microorganisms or inhibit their growth.

Anticoagulant—prevents clotting of the blood.

Antidepressant—helps to control depression.

Antidiabetic—regulates blood sugar levels.

Antifungal—destroys or controls fungus.

Antigout—controls symptoms of gout.

Antihypertensive—controls high BP.

Antimicrobial—kills or inhibits the growth of microorganisms.

Antimigraine—prevents or controls migraine headaches.

Antineoplastic—prevents the spread of neoplasms or malignant cells.

Antiprotozoal—kills protozoa.

Antipruritic—relieves itching.

Antitussive—helps to suppress coughing.

Antiviral—helps to prevent or control the spread of viruses.

Common Prescribed and Over-the-Counter Medications

Herbal Agents	Sometimes Used for
Ginkgo or *Ginkgo biloba*	Dementia, poor circulation to the legs, ringing in the ears
St. John's wort	Depression
Echinacea	Prevention and treatment of common cold
Garlic	High cholesterol
Ginger root	Nausea and vomiting
Saw palmetto	Swollen prostate
Hawthorn leaf or flower	Heart failure
Evening primrose oil	Premenstrual syndrome
Feverfew leaf	Migraine prevention
Valerian root	Insomnia

Beta blocker—prevents beta receptor site stimulation.
Blood glucose regulator—controls blood sugar levels.
Bronchodilator—opens up the constricted bronchial tree.
Calcium channel blocker—inhibits the transfer of calcium in smooth muscle cells.
Cephalosporin—a type of antibiotic.
CNS stimulant—stimulates activity of brain and spinal cord.
Contraceptive—prevents conception or sperm and egg uniting.
Coronary vasodilator—dilates the coronary vessels.
Corticosteroid—adrenal cortex steroid used for anti-inflammatory purposes.

Common Prescribed and Over-the-Counter Medications

Decongestant—relieves congestion of mucous membranes.

Diuretic—helps the body off-load water by stimulating kidneys.

Electrolytes—solutions that contain electrically charged ions used by the body.

Expectorant—promotes discharge of mucus from the respiratory tract.

Hormones—replace or alter endocrine system function.

NSAID (nonsteroidal anti-inflammatory drug)—controls muscular inflammation and pain.

Penicillin—commonly used antibiotic substance.

Progestin—female sex steroid hormone.

Sedative hypnotic—relaxes, calms, or tranquilizes a patient.

Skeletal muscle relaxant—calms muscle shaking, twitching, and spasm.

Sulfonamide—a type of antibiotic.

Tetracycline—a type of antibiotic.

Vitamins—substances found in foods that are necessary for body functions.

➤ THE "MEDS"

Accolate—bronchodilator
acetaminophen—analgesic, antipyretic
acetaminophen codeine phosphate—analgesic
acetaminophen hydrocodone bitartrate—analgesic
acetaminophen oxycodone hydrochloride—analgesic
acetaminophen propoxyphene napsylate—analgesic
acyclovir—antiviral
Adalat—antihypertensive
Adapin—antidepressant, antianxiety
albuterol—bronchodilator, antiasthmatic
Aldomet—antihypertensive
allopurinol—antigout
alprazolam—antianxiety, sedative hypnotic
amantadine—Parkinson's med
aminophylline—bronchodilator
amitriptyline—antidepressant
amoxapine—antidepressant
amoxicillin—penicillin, antibiotic
Amoxil—penicillin, antibiotic
Anacin-3—analgesic
Anafranil—antidepressant
Anaprox—analgesic, NSAID, antiarthritic
Anaprox DS—analgesic, antiarthritic, NSAID
Antivert—antihistimine, vertigo, motion sickness
Apresoline—antihypertensive
Aricept—Alzheimer's med
Aristocort—corticosteroid, antiasthmatic, sulfonamide
Asendin—antidepressant
aspirin—analgesic
Astramorph/PF—analgesic
Atarax—antihistimine, antipruritic, sedative

atenolol—antianginal, antihypertensive, beta blocker
Ativan—antianxiety, sedative hypnotic
Aventyl—antidepressant
Axert—migraine
Azmacort—inhaled corticosteroid, antiasthmatic

Bactrim—sulfonamide, antimicrobial
Barbita—anticonvulsant
benzonatate—antitussant
Bextra—analgesic
Brethaire—bronchodilator
Brethine—bronchodilator
Bricanyl—bronchodilator
Bronkometer—bronchodilator
Bronkosol—bronchodilator
bupropion—antidepressant

Calan—antiarrhythmic, antihypertensive
Calan SR—antiarrhythmic, antihypertensive
Capoten—antihypertensive, ACE inhibitor
captopril—antihypertensive, ACE inhibitor
carisoprodol—skeletal muscle relaxant
carbamazepine—anticonvulsant
Catapres—antihypertensive
Celexa—antidepressant
cephalexin—antibiotic, antimicrobial
chlorpropamide—antidiabetic
Cialis—erectile dysfunction
cimetidine—acid/peptic disorder
clomipramine—antidepressant
clonazepama—anticonvulsant
clonidine—antihypertensive

Common Prescribed and Over-the-Counter Medications

codeine—analgesic
codeine phosphate promethazine hydrochloride—antitussive, expectorant
Coreg—antiarrhythmic
Coumadin—anticoagulant
Cycrin—antineoplastic, progestin, contraceptive
cyclobenzaprine hydrochloride—skeletal muscle relaxant

Darvocet-N—analgesic
Darvon—analgesic
Deltasone—corticosteroid, antiarthritic, antineoplastic
Depakene—anticonvulsant
desipramine—antidepressant
Desyrel—antianxiety, antidepressant
DiaBeta—antidiabetic, blood glucose regulator
Diabinese—antidiabetic
diazepam—antianxiety, anticonvulsant, skeletal muscle relaxant
diclofenac—analgesic, antiarthritic, NSAID
digoxin—antiarrhythmic, cardiac glycoside
Dilantin—anticonvulsant
doxepin—antidepressant
doxepin hydrochloride—antianxiety, antidepressant
doxycycline—antibiotic, antimicrobial
Duramorph—analgesic
Dyazide—antihypertensive, diuretic
Dynacin—tetracycline

Ecotrin—analgesic
Effexor—antidepressant
Elavil—antidepressant
Elixophyllin—antiasthmatic

Common Prescribed and Over-the-Counter Medications

Emprin—analgesic
Epitol—anticonvulsant
Esidrix—antihypertensive
estrogen—hormone
Excedrin IS—analgesic

Fastin—anorexiant
Flagyl—antibacterial, antiprotozoal
Flexeril—skeletal muscle relaxant
fluoxetine—antidepressant
folic acid—vitamin
Folvite—anemia, vitamin
Frova—migraine
furosemide—antihypertensive, diuretic

gemfibrozil—antilipemic
glipizide—antidiabetic
Glucophage—antidiabetic
Glucotrol—blood glucose regulator
Glucotrol XL—blood glucose regulator
glyburide—antidiabetic, blood glucose regulator
Glynase Prestab—antidiabetic, blood glucose regulator
guaifenesin phenylpropanolamine hychloride—
antitussive, expectorant, decongestant
guanabenz—antihypertensive

Humulin—antidiabetic
hydralazine—antihypertensive
hydrochlorothiazide—antihypertensive
hydrochlorothiazide triamterene—antihypertensive,
diuretic

Hydro DIURIL—antihypertensive
hydroxyzine hydrochloride—antianxiety, antihistimine, antipruritic, sedative hypnotic

ibuprofen—NSAID, antiarthritic, analgesic, antipyretic
Imdur—antianginal, coronary vasodilator
imipramine hydrochloride—antidepressant
Imitrex—migraine
indapamide—antihypertensive, diuretic
Inderal—antianginal, antiarrhythmic, antihypertensive, antimigraine, beta blocker
Indocin—antiarthritic, antigout
indomethacin—antiarthritic, NSAID, antigout
insulin—antidiabetic
Ionamin—anorexiant
Ismo—antianginal, coronary vasodilator
isoetharine—bronchodilator
Isoptin—antiarrhythmic, antiarthritic, antianginal, antihypertensive, calcium channel blocker
Isoptin SR—antiarrhythmic, antiarthritic, antianginal, antihypertensive, calcium channel blocker
isosorbide mononitrate—antianginal, coronary vasodilator

Janimine—antidepressant

K-Dur—electrolyte, water balance, mineral
Keflex—cephalosporin
Kenalog—corticosteroid
Klonopin—anticonvulsant
K-Tab—electrolyte, water balance, mineral

Lanoxin—antiarrhythmic, cardiac glycoside
Lanoxicaps—antiarrhythmic, cardiac glycoside
Larotid—penicillin
Lasix—antihypertensive, diuretic
Levitra—erectile dysfunction
Lopid—antilipemic
Lopressor—antianginal, antihypertensive, beta blocker
Lopurin—antigout
lorazepam—antianxiety, sedative hypnotic
Lorcet—analgesic
Lozol—antihypertensive, diuretic
Luminal—antianxiety, anticonvulsant, sedative hypnotic, anticonvulsant

Maxzide—antihypertensive, diuretic
Mazepine—anticonvulsant
meclizine hydrochloride—antihistimine, vertigo, motion sickness
medroxyprogesterone acetate—contraceptive, progestin
metformin—antidiabetic
methyldopa—antihypertensive
methylphenidate hydrochloride—CNS stimulant
Meticorten—corticosteroids, antiarthritic
Metoclopramide hydrochloride—antiemetic, acid/peptic, motion sickness
metoprolol tartrate—antianginal, antihypertensive, beta blocker
metronidazole—antibacterial, antiprotozoal
Micro-K—electrolye, water balance
Micronase—antidiabetic, blood glucose regulator
Minocin—tetracycline

minocycline hydrochloride–tetracycline
Monoket–antianginal, coronary vasodilator
Motrin–analgesic, NSAID, antiarthritic, antipyretic
MS Contin–analgesic
Mysoline–anticonvulsant

nalbuphine–analgesic
Naprosyn–analgesic, antiarthritic, NSAID
naproxen–analgesic, antiarthritic, NSAID
Nasacort–corticosteroid, antiasthmatic
nefazodone–antidepressant
nifedipine–antihypertensive
Nitro-Bid–antianginal, antihypertensive, coronary vasodilator
Nitro-Dur–antianginal, antihypertensive, coronary vasodilator
nitroglycerin–antianginal, antihypertensive, coronary vasodilator
Nitrostat–antianginal
Nolvadex–antineoplastic, hormonal/biological response
Norpace–antidysrhythmic
Norpramin–antidepressant
nortriptyline hydrochloride–antidepressant
Novolin–antidiabetic
Novoprofen–analgesic
NPH insulin–antidiabetic
Nubain–analgesic
Nuprin–analgesic

Oretic–antihypertensive
Orinase–antidiabetic

Common Prescribed and Over-the-Counter Medications

Pamelor—antidepressant
Pamprin-IB—analgesic
Pamelor—antidepressant
Panadol—analgesic
paroxetine—antidepressant
Paxil—antidepressant
penicillin V potassium—penicillin, antibiotic
Pen-Vee K—penicillin, antibiotic
Percocet—analgesic
Pertofrane—antidepressant
Phenergan—antiemetic, antitussive, expectorant
Phenergan with codeine—antitussive, expectorant
phenobarbital—anticonvulsant, antianxiety, sedative
hypnotic
Phentermine hydrochloride—anorexiant
phenytoin—anticonvulsant
potassium chloride—electrolyte, water balance,
vitamin, mineral
prednisone—corticosteroid, antiarthritic
primidone—anticonvulsant
procainamide—antiarrhythmic
Procan SR—antiarrhythmic
Procardia—antihypertensive
progesterone—hormone
promethazine hydrochloride—antiemetic, antitussive,
expectorant
Pronestyl—antiarrhythmic
propoxyphene—analgesic
propranolol hydrochloride—antianginal,
antiarrhythmic, antihypertensive, antimigraine,
beta blocker
Protostat—antibacterial, antiprotozoal

protriptyline—antidepressant
Proventil—bronchodilator, antiasthmatic
Proventil Inhaler—antiasthmatic, bronchodilator
Provera—contraceptive, progestin
Prozac—antidepressant

Reglan—antiemetic, acid/peptic
Relafen—NSAID
Relapax—migraine
Restoril—sedative hypnotic
Ritalin—CNS stimulant
Ritalin-SR—CNS stimulant
Roxanol—analgesic
Rufen—NSAID, antiarthritic, analgesic, antipyretic

Septra—sulfonamide, antimicrobial
sertraline—antidepressant
Sinequam—antidepressant, antianxiety
Sinequan Concentrate—antidepressant
Singulair—bronchodilator
Slo-Bid—antiasthmatic
Slo-Phyllin—antiasthmatic
Slow-K—electrolyte, water balance, vitamin, mineral
Solfoton—anticonvulsant
Soma—skeletal muscle relaxant
sulfamethoxazole trimethoprim—sulfonamide,
antimicrobial

Tagamet—acid/peptic disorder
tamoxifen citrate—antineoplastic, hormonal/biological
response
Tegretol—anticonvulsant

Common Prescribed and Over-the-Counter Medications

temazepam—sedative hypnotic
Tempra—analgesic, antipyretic
Ten-K—electrolyte, water balance, vitamin, mineral
Tenormin—antianginal, antihypertensive, beta blocker
terbutaline—bronchodilator
Tessalon Perles—antitussant
Theo-24—antiasthmatic
Theo-Dur—antiasthmatic, bronchodilator
theophylline—bronchodilator, antiasthmatic
Tofranil—antidepressant
tolbutamde—antidiabetic
Toprol XL—antidysrhythmic
topramax—anticonvulsant
T-Phyl—bronchodilator
trazodone hydrochloride—analgesic, antianxiety, antidepressant, antiarthritic
Triadapin—antidepressant
triamcinolone acetonide—corticosteroid, sulfonamide, antiasthmatic
trimipramine—antidepressant
Trimox—penicillin, antibiotic
Tripramine—antidepressant
Tylenol—analgesic, antipyretic
Tylenol with Codeine—analgesic
Tylox—analgesic

Uniphyl—bronchodilator

Valium—antianxiety, anticonvulsant, skeletal muscle relaxant
valproic acid—anticonvulsant
V-Cillin K—penicillin

Ventolin—bronchodilator
verapamil—antiarrhythmic, antihypertensive
Verelan—antiarrhythmic, antianginal, antiarthritic, antihypertensive, calcium channel blocker
Viagra—erectile dysfunction
Vibramycin—tetracycline, antibiotic
Vicodin—analgesic
Vioxx—analgesic
Vivactil—antidepressant
Voltaren—analgesic, antiarthritic, NSAID

warfarin sodium—anticoagulant
Wellbutrin—antidepressant
Wymox—penicillin, antibiotic
Wytensin—antihypertensive

Xanax—antianxiety, sedative

Zoloft—antidepressant
Zonalon—antianxiety, antidepressant
Zovirax—antiviral
Zyloprim—antigout

➤ AIDS (ACQUIRED IMMUNE DEFICIENCY SYNDROME)

Mode of Transmission—infected blood via intravenous drug use, unprotected sexual contact, blood transfusions, or (rarely) accidental needle sticks. Mothers also may pass HIV to their unborn children.
Incubation—several months or years.

➤ CHICKENPOX (VARICELLA)

Mode of Transmission—airborne droplets. Can also be spread by contact with open sores.
Incubation—11 to 21 days.

➤ GERMAN MEASLES (RUBELLA)

Mode of Transmission—airborne droplets. Mothers may pass the disease to unborn children.
Incubation—10 to 12 days.

➤ VIRAL HEPATITIS

Mode of Transmission—blood, stool, or other body fluids, or contaminated objects.
Incubation—weeks to months, depending on type.

➤ MENINGITIS, BACTERIAL

Mode of Transmission—oral and nasal secretions.
Incubation—2 to 10 days.

➤ MUMPS

Mode of Transmission—droplets of saliva or objects contaminated by saliva.
Incubation—14 to 24 days.

➤ PNEUMONIA, BACTERIAL AND VIRAL

Mode of Transmission—oral and nasal droplets and secretions.
Incubation—several days.

➤ SEVERE ACUTE RESPIRATORY SYNDROME (SARS-CoV DISEASE)

Severe acute respiratory syndrome is a viral respiratory illness caused by a coronavirus, called SARS-associated coronavirus (SARS-CoV). First reported in Asia in February 2003, the illness spread over the next few months to more than two dozen countries in North America, South America, Europe, and Asia before the global outbreak was contained.

According to the CDC, safe work practices to prevent transmission of SARS-CoV for EMS providers would include:

• Avoid touching your face with contaminated gloves.

• Avoid unnecessary touching of surface in the ambulance.

• Arrange for the receiving facility staff to meet the patient at the ambulance door to limit the need for EMS providers to enter the ED in contaminated PPE.

(continued)

- If possible, remove and discard PPE after transferring the patient at the ED and perform handwashing.
- Treat used disposable PPE as medical waste.
- Clean the ambulance used to transport a SARS patient to prevent SARS-CoV transmission according to your service's exposure control plan.
- Additional information can be obtained by visiting www.cdc.gov/ncidod/sars or calling the CDC public response hotline at (888) 246-2675.

➤ STAPHYLOCOCCAL SKIN INFECTION

Mode of Transmission—direct contact with infected wounds or sores or with contaminated objects.
Incubation—several days.

➤ TUBERCULOSIS (TB)

Mode of Transmission—respiratory secretions, airborne, or on contaminated objects.
Incubation—2 to 6 weeks.

➤ WHOOPING COUGH (PERTUSSIS)

Mode of Transmission—respiratory secretions or airborne droplets.
Incubation—6 to 20 days.

➤ AIRBORNE INFECTION
(such as TB)

- You have transported a patient who is infected with a life-threatening airborne disease, but you are not aware that the patient is infected.

- After the medical facility diagnoses the disease in the patient, they must notify your designated infectious disease officer within 48 hours.

- Your officer then notifies you that you have been exposed.

- Your employer arranges for you to be evaluated, with a follow-up by a doctor or appropriate other health care professional.

➤ **BLOOD-BORNE INFECTION**
  (such as HIV or HBV)

- You have come into contact with blood and body fluids of a patient, and you wonder if that patient is infected with a life-threatening disease such as HIV or HBV.

- You seek immediate medical attention and document the incident for worker's compensation.

- You ask your designated officer (DO) to determine if you have been exposed to an infectious disease.

- Your DO must gather information and, if warranted, consult the medical facility to which the patient was transported.

- The medical facility must gather information and report findings to your DO within 48 hours.

- Your DO notifies you of the findings.

- Your employer arranges for you to be evaluated, with a follow-up by a doctor or appropriate other health care professional.

Standard Abbreviations

=—equal.
+—positive.
-—negative.
>—greater than.
<—less than.
×—times or multiply.
@—at.
Δ—change.

ā—before.
AAA—abdominal aortic aneurysm.
AAL—anterior axillary line.
ABCs—airway, breathing, circulation.
Abd—abdominal.
ADD—attention deficit disorder.
ADHD—attention deficit hyperactivity disorder.
AED—automated external defibrillator.
AIDS—acquired immune deficiency syndrome.
ALS—advanced life support.
AMA—against medical advice.
AMI—acute myocardial infarction.
AMS—altered mental status.
A/O—alert and oriented.
A/P—anterior and posterior.
APE—acute pulmonary edema.
APGAR—appearance, pulse, grimace, activity, respiratory effort.
ASHD—arteriosclerotic heart disease.
ATV—automatic transport ventilator.
AVPU—alert, verbally responsive, painful response, unresponsive.

BAC—blood alcohol content.
BG—blood glucose.
b.i.d.—twice daily.
BLS—basic life support.
b.m.—bowel movement.
BMV—bag-mask ventilation.
BP—blood pressure.
bpm—beats per minute.
BSA—body surface area.
BSI—body substance isolation.
BVM—bag-valve-mask resuscitator.

c̄—with.
CABG—coronary artery bypass graft.
CAD—coronary artery disease.
c/c—chief complaint.
cc—cubic centimeter.
CCU—critical care unit.
CHF—congestive heart failure.
CISM\D—critical incident stress management\ Debriefing.
CNS—central nervous system.
c/o—complained of.
CO—carbon monoxide.
CO_2—carbon dioxide.
COPD—chronic obstructive pulmonary disease.
CPR—cardiopulmonary resuscitation.
CSF—cerebrospinal fluid.
CT—computerized tomography.
CUPS—critical, unstable, potentially unstable, stable.
CVA—cerebrovascular accident.

Standard Abbreviations

DCAP-BTLS—deformities, contusions, abrasions, punctures, burns, tenderness, lacerations, swelling.
D5W—5 percent dextrose in water.
DAN—Diver's Alert Network.
d/c—discontinue.
DKA—diabetic ketoacidosis.
DNAR—do not attempt resuscitation.
DNR—do not resuscitate.
DOA—dead on arrival.
DOB—date of birth.
Dr.—doctor.
DTs—delirium tremens.
Dx—diagnosis.

ECG—electrocardiogram; also called EKG.
ED—emergency department.
EEG—electroencephalogram.
EENT—ears, eyes, nose, throat.
EID—esophageal intubation device.
EMD—emergency medical dispatch.
EMS—emergency medical services.
EMT—emergency medical technician.
EMT-B—EMT-Basic.
EMT-I—EMT-Intermediate.
EMT-P—EMT-Paramedic.
EOA—esophageal obturator airway.
EPI—epinephrine.
ER—emergency room.
ET—endotracheal tube.
ETA—estimated time of arrival.
EtCO$_2$—end-tidal carbon dioxide.
EtOH—ethyl alcohol.

Standard Abbreviations

FBAO—foreign-body airway obstruction.
FROPVD—flow-restricted oxygen-powered ventilation device.
FUO—fever of unknown origin.
fx—fracture.

GCS—Glasgow Coma Score.
GI—gastrointestinal.
GSW—gunshot wound.
gtt—drops.
GU—genitourinary.
GYN—gynecology.

H—hour.
HBV—hepatitis B virus.
HIV—human immunodeficiency virus.
Hx—history.

ICP—intracranial pressure.
ICS—incident command system.
ICU—intensive care unit.
IM—intramuscular.
IMS—incident management system.
IO—intraosseous.
IUD—intrauterine device.
IV—intravenous.
IVP—intravenous push.

JVD—jugular vein distention.

KED—Kendrick Extrication Device.
kg—kilogram.
KVO—keep vein open.

L—liter.
L.—left.
LLQ—left lower quadrant (of abdomen).
LMA—laryngeal mask airway.
LOC—loss of (or level of) consciousness.
LPN—licensed practical nurse.
LR—lactated Ringer's.
LUQ—left upper quadrant (of abdomen).

MAST—military anti-shock trousers.
MCI—multiple-casualty incident.
MD—physician.
mg—milligram.
MI—myocardial infarction.
ml—milliliter.
mm—millimeter.
mmHg—millimeters mercury.
MOI—mechanism of injury.
MPDS—medical priority dispatch system.
MRI—magnetic resonance imaging.
MS-ABC—mental status, airway, breathing, circulation.
MVA—motor-vehicle accident.
MVC—motor vehicle crash.

N/A—not applicable.
NG—nasogastric.
NIMS—National Incident Management System.
NKA—no known allergies.
NKDA—no known drug allergies.
NPA—nasopharyngeal (nasal) airway.
NRB—nonrebreather face mask.
NS—normal saline.

NSR—normal sinus rhythm.
NTG—nitroglycerin.
N/V—nausea and vomiting.

O₂—oxygen.
OB/GYN—obstetrics and gynecology.
OD—overdose.
OPA—oropharyngeal (oral) airway.
OPQRST—onset, provocation, quality, referral, radiation, region, severity, time.
OR—operating room.
O.T.C.—over the counter.
oz.—ounce.

P—pulse.
P.A.—physician assistant.
PASG—pneumatic anti-shock garment.
PCR—prehospital care report.
PE—physical exam.
PEA—pulseless electrical activity.
PEARL—pupils equal and reactive to light.
PFD—personal floatation device.
PIAA—personal injury auto accident.
PID—pelvic inflammatory disease.
PMH—past medical history.
PMS—pulses, motor ability, and sensory response; premenstrual syndrome.
p.o.—by mouth.
PPE—personal protective equipment.
p.r.n.—as needed.
PSAP—public safety access point.

p.s.i.—pounds per square inch.
pt—patient; pint.

q.—every.
q.d.—every day.
q.h.—every hour.
q.i.d.—four times a day.
qod—every other day.

R.—right.
RBC—red blood cells.
RLQ—right lower quadrant (of abdomen).
RMA—refused medical assistance.
RN—registered nurse.
r/o—rule out.
R.O.M.—range of motion.
ROSC—return of spontaneous circulation.
RPM—respirations, pulse, mental status.
RR—respiratory rate.
RUQ—right upper quadrant (of abdomen).
R$_x$—prescription.

s̄—without.
SA—sinoatrial.
SAMPLE—symptoms, allergies, meds, pertinent past medical hx, last oral intake, events leading up to.
s.c.—subcutaneous. Also called sq.
SIDS—sudden infant death syndrome.
SL—sublingual.
SOB—shortness of breath.
sq.—subcutaneous. Also called s.c.

START—simple triage and rapid transport.
S.T.D.—sexually transmitted disease.

TB—tuberculosis.
TIA—transient ischemic attack.
t.i.d.—three times a day.
TKO—to keep open.
TOT—turned over to.

URI—upper respiratory infection.
UTI—urinary tract infection.

VD—venereal disease.
VF—ventricular fibrillation.
V.S.—vital signs.

w/—with.
WBC—white blood cells.
WNL—within normal limits.
w/o—without.

y/o—year old.

Standard Terms and Planes

abduction—movement away from the body's midline.
adduction—movement toward the body's midline.
afferent—conducting toward a structure.
anatomical position—body is erect with arms down at sides, palms front.
anterior—the front surface of the body.
anterior to—in front of.

caudad—toward the tail.
cephalad—toward the head.
circumduction—circular movement of a part.
coronal plane—an imaginary plane that passes through body from side to side and divides it into front and back sections. Also called frontal plane.
craniad—toward the cranium.

deep—situated remote from surface.
distal—situated away from point of origin.
dorsal—pertaining to the back surface of body.
dorsiflexion—bending backward.

efferent—conducting away from a structure.
elevation—raising a body part.
extension—stretching or moving jointed parts into or toward a straight condition.
external—situated outside.

flexion—bending or moving jointed parts closer together.
frontal plane—an imaginary plane that passes through body from side to side and divides it into front and back sections. Also called coronal plane.

inferior—situated below.
internal—situated inside.

lateral—situated away from the body's midline.
lateral rotation—rotating outward away from the body's midline.
left lateral recumbent—lying down or reclining on left side.

mediad—toward the midline of body.
medial—situated toward body's midline.
medial rotation—rotating inward toward body's midline.
midsagittal plane—an imaginary plane that passes through body from front to back and divides it into right and left halves.

palmar—concerning inner surface of hand.
peripheral—away from a central structure.
plantar—concerning the sole of the foot.
posterior—pertaining to back surface of body.
posterior to—situated behind.
pronation—lying face downward or turning hand so palm faces downward or backward.
prone—lying face down and flat.
protraction—a pushing forward of part of body, such as mandible.
proximal—situated nearest the point of origin.

recumbent—lying down, reclining.
retraction—a drawing back, as of the tongue.

right lateral recumbent—lying down on right side.
rotation—turning around an axis.

sagittal plane—an imaginary plane parallel to medial plane; passes through body from front to back and divides body into right and left sections.
superficial—situated near surface.
superior—situated above.
supination—lying face upward or turning hand so palm faces forward or upward.
supine—lying down flat on back and face up.

transverse plane—an imaginary plane that passes through body and divides it into upper and lower sections.

ventral—front surface of body.

Prefixes are followed by a dash. Suffixes are preceded by a dash. All others are combining forms, which usually have a slash and a vowel after the word root.

a- not, without, lacking, deficient.
ab- away from.
-able capable of.
abdomin/o abdomen.
ac- to, toward, pertaining to.
acou hear.
acr/o extremity, top, peak.
acu- with a needle.
ad- to, toward.
aden/o gland.
adip/o fat.
-aemia blood.
aer/o air.
-aesthesia sensation.
-algesia painful.
-algia painful.
af- to.
algi- pain.
all- other.
ambi- both sides.
ambly/o dim, dull, lazy.
amph- on both sides, around both.
amyl/o starch.
an- without, negative.
ana- upward, again, backward, excess.
andr/o man, male.
angi/o blood vessel, duct.
anis/o unequal.

ankyl/o   stiff.
ant-   against, opposed to, preventing.
ante-   before, in front of.
antero-   from front to.
anti-   against, opposed to, preventing.
ap-   to.
apo-   separation, derivation from.
-arium   place for something.
arteri/o   artery.
arthr/o   joint, articulation.
articul/o   joint.
as-   to.
-ase   enzyme.
at-   to.
audi/o   hearing.
aur/o   ear.
aut/o   self.

bi-   two, twice, double, both.
bis-   twice, double.
bi/o   life.
blephar/o   eyelid.
brachi/o   upper arm.
brady-   slow.
bronch/o   larger air passages of lungs.
bucc/o   cheek.

cac/o   bad, evil.
calc/o   stone.
calcane/o   heel.
calor/o   heat.
cancr/o   cancer.

capit/o   head.

caps/o   container.

carcin/o   cancer.

cardi/o   heart.

carp/o   wrist bone.

cat-   down, lower, under, against, along with.

cata-   down, lower, under, against, along with.

-cele   tumor, a cyst, hernia.

celi/o   abdomen.

cent   hundred.

-centesis   perforation, puncture, or tapping with a needle.

cephal/o   head.

cerebr/o   cerebrum.

cervic/o   neck, cervix.

cheil/o   lip.

cheir/o   hand.

chil/o   lip.

chir/o   hand.

chlor/o   green.

chol/e   bile, gall.

chondr/o   cartilage.

chrom/o   color.

chromat/o   color.

chron/o   time.

-cid   cut, kill, fall.

-cide   causing death.

circum-   around.

-cis   cut, kill, fall.

clysis   irrigation.

co-   with.

col- with.

col/o colon, large intestine.

colp/o vagina.

com- with, together.

con- together.

contra- against, opposite.

cor/e pupil.

cost/o rib.

crani/o skull.

cry/o cold.

crypt/o hide, cover, conceal.

cyan/o blue.

cyst/o urinary bladder, cyst, sac of fluid.

-cyte cell.

cyt/o cell.

dacry/o tear.

dactyl/o finger, toe.

de- down, from, not.

deca- ten.

deci- tenth.

demi- half.

dent/o tooth.

derm/o skin.

dermat/o skin.

dextr/o right.

di- twice, double.

dia- through, across, apart.

dipl/o double, twin, twice.

dips/o thirst.

dis- to free, to undo.

Word Parts

dors/o back.
-dynia pain.
dys- bad, difficult, abnormal, incomplete.

-ectasia dilation or enlargement of organ or part.
ecto- outer, outside of.
-ectomy the surgical removal of organ/part.
ef- out.
electr/o electric.
emesis vomiting.
-emia condition of the blood.
en- in, into, within.
encephal/o brain.
end- within.
endo- within.
ent- within, inner.
ento- within, inner.
enter/o small intestine.
ep- over, on, upon.
epi- over, on, upon.
erythr/o red.
-esthesia feeling, sensation.
eu- good, well, normal, healthy.
ex- out of, away from.
exo- outside, outward.
extra- on the outside, beyond, in addition to.

faci/o face, surface.
febr/i fever.
-ferent bear, carry.
fibr/o fiber, filament.
fore- before, in front of.

Word Parts

-form shape.
-fugal moving away, passing from.
-fuge one that drives away.

galact/o milk.
gangli/o mass, knot.
-gaster stomach, belly.
gastr/o stomach.
gen/o come into being, originate.
-genesis production or origin.
-genic giving rise to, originating in.
gloss/o tongue.
glyc/o sweet.
gnath/o jaw.
gnos/o knowledge.
-gog to make flow.
-gogue to make flow.
-gram drawing, written record.
-graph an instrument for recording activity of an organ.
-graphy the recording of the activity of an organ.
gynec/o woman.

hem/a blood.
hem/o blood.
hemat/o blood.
hemi- one-half.
hepat/o liver.
heter/o other, dissimilarity.
hidr/o sweat.
hist/o tissue.
hol/o all, entire, total, complete.
hom/o same, similar, unchanging constant.

home/o same, similar, unchanging constant.
hyal/o glass.
hydr/o water, fluid.
hyp- under.
hyper- beyond, normal, excessive.
hypn/o sleep.
hypo- below normal, deficient, under, beneath.
hyster/o uterus, womb.

-iasis condition, pathological state.
iatr/o healer, physician.
-ible capable of.
-id in a state, condition of.
idio- peculiar, separate, distinct.
il- negative, prefix.
ile/o ileum.
ili/o ilium.
im- negative, prefix.
in- in, into, within.
infra- beneath, below.
inter- between.
intra- within.
intro- within, into.
irid/o iris.
ischi/o ischium.
-ism condition, theory.
-ismus abnormal condition.
iso- same, equal, alike.
-itis inflammation.
-ize to treat by special method.

juxta near, nearby.

Word Parts

karyo nucleus, nut.
kata- down, against.
kera- horn, indicates hardness.
kerat/o cornea.
kinesi/o movement, motion.
-kinesis motion.

labi/o lip.
lact/o milk.
lal/o talk.
lapar/o flank, abdomen, abdominal wall.
laryng/o larynx.
later/o side.
lept/o thin, small, soft.
leuc/o white.
leuk/o white.
lingu/o tongue.
lip/o fat.
lith/o stone.
-logist a person who studies.
log/o speak.
-logy study of.
lumb/o loin.
lymph/o lymph.
-lysis destruction.

macr/o large, long.
mal- bad, poor, evil.
malac/o a softening.
mamm/o breast.
-mania mental aberration.
mast/o breast.

medi/o middle.
mega- large.
megal/o large.
-megaly an enlargement.
melan/o dark, black.
men/o month.
mes/o middle.
meta- change, transformation, exchange.
-meter measure.
metr/o uterus.
micr/o small.
mi/o less, smaller.
mon/o single, only, sole.
morph/o form.
multi- many, much.
myc/o fungus.
mycet/o fungus.
my/o muscle.
myel/o marrow, also refers to spinal cord.
myx/o mucus, slimelike.

narc/o stupor, numbness.
nas/o nose.
ne/o new.
necr/o corpse.
nephr/o kidney.
neur/o nerve.
niter- nitrogen.
nitro- nitrogen.
noct/i night.
non- not.
norm/o rule, order, normal.

Word Parts

nucleo- nucleus.
null/i none.
nyct/o night.

ob- against, in front of, toward.
ocul/o eye.
odont/o tooth.
-oid shape, form, resemblance.
olig/o few, deficient, scanty.
-oma tumor, swelling.
omo- shoulder.
o/o -egg.
onych/o nail.
oophor/o ovary.
opisth- backward.
-opsy a viewing.
opthalm/o eye.
opt/o sight, vision.
optic/o sight, vision.
or/o mouth.
orch/o testicle.
orchid/o testicle.
-orium place for something.
orth/o straight, upright.
os- mouth, bone.
-osis process, an abnormal condition.
oste/o bone.
-ostomosis to furnish with a mouth or outlet.
-otomy cutting.
ot/o ear.
ovari/o ovary.
ov/i egg.

ov/o egg.
oxy- sharp, acid.

pachy- thicken.
palat/o palate.
pan- all entire, every.
para- beside, beyond, accessory to, apart from, against.
path/o disease.
-pathy disease of a part.
-penia an abnormal reduction.
peps/o digestion.
pept/o digestion.
per- throughout, completely, extremely.
peri- around, surrounding.
-pexy fixation.
phag/o ear.
pharyng/o throat.
phas/o speech.
phil/o like, have an affinity for.
phleb/o vein.
-phobia fear, dread.
phon/o sound.
phor/o bear, carry.
phot/o light.
phren/o diaphragm.
-phylaxis protection.
physi/o nature.
pil/o hair.
-plasia development, formation.
-plasm to mold.
-plasty surgical repair.

Word Parts

-plegia paralysis, a stroke.
pleur/o rib, side, pleura.
plur more.
pnea- breath, breathing.
pneum/o lung, air, breath.
pneumat/o air, breath.
pneumon/o lung.
pod/o foot.
-poies is formation.
poly- much, many.
post- after, behind.
pre- before.
pro- before, in front of.
proto first.
proct/o anus.
pseud/o false.
psych/o mind, soul.
-ptosis abnormal dropping/sagging of part.
pulmon/o lung.
py/o pus.
pyel/o renal pelvis.
pyr/o fire, fever.

quadri- four.

rach/i spine.
radio- ray, radiation.
re- back, against, contrary.
rect/o rectum.
ren/o kidneys.
retro- located behind, backward.
-rhage hemorrhage, flow.

-rhaphy   a suturing or stitching.
-rhea   to flow, indicates discharge.
rhin/o   nose.
-rrhage   abnormal discharge.
-rrhagia   hemorrhage from organ/body part.
-rrhea   flowing or discharge.

sacchar   sugar.
sacr/o   sacrum.
salping-   a tube, relating to a fallopian tube.
sanguin/o   blood.
sarc/o   flesh.
schiz/o   split.
scler/o   hardening.
-sclerosis   hardening condition.
scoli/o   twisted, crooked.
-scope   an instrument for observing.
-scopy   to see.
-sect   cut.
semi-   one-half, partly.
seps/o   infection.
sept/o   infection.
somat/o   body.
son/o   sound.
spermat/o   sperm, semen.
sphygm/o   pulse.
splen/o   spleen.
-stasis   stopping, controlling.
sten/o   narrow.
stere/o   solid, three-dimensional.
steth/o   chest.
sthen/o   strength.

-stomy surgically creating a new opening.
sub- under, near, almost, moderately.
super- above, excess.
supra- above, over.
sym- joined together, with.
syn- joined together, with.

tachy- fast.
tele- distant, far.
tetra- four.
therm/o heat.
thio- sulfur.
thorac/o chest cavity.
thromb/o clot, lump.
thyro- thyroid gland.
-tome surgical instrument for cutting.
-tomy surgical operation on organ/body part.
top/o place.
trache/o trachea.
trans- through, across, beyond.
tri- three.
trich/o hair.
-tripsy surgical crushing.
troph/o nourish.

ultra- beyond, excess.
uni- one.
ur/o urine.
ureter/o ureter.
urethr/o urethra.
-uria relating to urine.

vas/o   vessel, duct.
ven/o   vein.
ventr/o   belly, cavity.
vesic/o   blister, bladder.
viscer/o   internal organ.

xanth/o   yellow.
xen/o   stranger.
xer/o   dry.

zo/o   animal life.

This Pocket Reference Belongs to:

_____

Important Phone Numbers

911 Dispatch Center _____

American Red Cross _____

CHEMTREC Emergency 1-800-424-9300

CHEMTREC Nonemergency 1-800-262-8200

CISD Team _____

Child Abuse Hotline _____

Confined Space Rescue

Diver's Alert Network 1-919-684-8111 or 1-919-684-4DAN(collect)

HAZMAT Team _____

High-Angle Rescue _____

Hospital _____

Hospital _____

Hospital _____

Hospital _____

Medical Examiner / Coroner _____

Poison Control Center 1-800-222-1222

Water Rescue Team _____

Ambulance-to-Hospital Radio Report

- Unit identification (Ambulance # _____)
- Level of provider. _____
- Estimated time of arrival (ETA). _____
- Patient's age and sex. _____
- Chief complaint (why the patient called ambulance). _____
- Brief, pertinent history of present illness or injury. _____
- Major past illnesses. _____
- Mental status (AVPU). _____
- Baseline vital signs. _____
- Pertinent findings of physical exam. _____
- Emergency medical care given. _____
- Response to emergency medical care. _____
- Does medical direction have any questions or orders? _____

NOTE: *There are a number of local formats for radio reports, which may differ somewhat from the example above. However, they all adhere to the same basic principles. They should follow a logical order, be concise, and paint a picture of patient's problem and priorities for hospital care.*